PALEO DIET COOKCOOK 2022

DELICIOUS AND EASY RECIPES FOR BEGINNERS

JENNY KURZ

Table of Contents

Smoked Baby Back Ribs with Apple-Mustard Mop Sauce 9
Ribs 9
Sauce 9
Oven BBQ Country-Style Pork Ribs with Fresh Pineapple Slaw 12
Spicy Pork Goulash 14
Goulash 14
Cabbage 14
Italian Sausage Meatballs Marinara with Sliced Fennel and Onion Sauté 16
Meatballs 16
Marinara 16
Pork-Stuffed Zucchini Boats with Basil and Pine Nuts 18
Curried Pork and Pineapple "Noodle" Bowls with Coconut Milk and Herbs 20
Spicy Grilled Pork Patties with Tangy Cucumber Salad 22
Zucchini-Crust Pizza with Sun-Dried Tomato Pesto, Sweet Peppers, and Italian Sausage 24
Smoked Lemon-Coriander Lamb Leg with Grilled Asparagus 26
Lamb Hot Pot 28
Lamb Stew with Celery-Root Noodles 30
Frenched Lamb Chops with Pomegranate-Date Chutney 32
Chutney 32
Lamb Chops 32
Chimichurri Lamb Loin Chops with Sautéed Radicchio Slaw 34
Ancho-and-Sage-Rubbed Lamb Chops with Carrot-Sweet Potato Remoulade 36
Lamb Chops with Shallot, Mint, and Oregano Rub 38
Lamb 38
Salad 38
Garden-Stuffed Lamb Burgers with Red Pepper Coulis 40
Red Pepper Coulis 40
Burgers 40
Double-Oregano Lamb Kabobs with Tzatziki Sauce 43
Lamb Kabobs 43
Tzatziki Sauce 43

Roast Chicken with Saffron and Lemon 45

Spatchcocked Chicken with Jicama Slaw 47

Chicken.. 47

Slaw 47

Roasted Chicken Hindquarters with Vodka, Carrot, and Tomato Sauce 50

Poulet Rôti and Rutabaga Frites 52

Triple-Mushroom Coq au Vin with Chive Mashed Rutabagas 54

Peach-Brandy-Glazed Drumsticks 56

Peach-Brandy Glaze.. 56

Chile-Marinated Chicken with Mango-Melon Salad.. 58

Chicken.. 58

Salad 58

Tandoori-Style Chicken Legs with Cucumber Raita 61

Chicken.. 61

Cucumber Raita... 61

Curried Chicken Stew with Root Vegetables, Asparagus, and Green Apple-Mint Relish.. 63

Grilled Chicken Paillard Salad with Raspberries, Beets, and Roasted Almonds 65

Broccoli Rabe-Stuffed Chicken Breasts with Fresh Tomato Sauce and Caesar Salad 67

Grilled Chicken Shawarma Wraps with Spiced Vegetables and Pine Nut Dressing . 69

Oven-Braised Chicken Breasts with Mushrooms, Garlic-Mashed Cauliflower, and Roasted Asparagus 71

Thai-Style Chicken Soup 73

Lemon and Sage Roasted Chicken with Endive... 75

Chicken with Scallions, Watercress, and Radishes.. 78

Chicken Tikka Masala 80

Ras el Hanout Chicken Thighs 83

Star Fruit Adobo Chicken Thighs over Braised Spinach.. 85

Chicken-Poblano Cabbage Tacos with Chipotle Mayo 87

Chicken Stew with Baby Carrots and Bok Choy 89

Cashew-Orange Chicken and Sweet Pepper Stir-Fry in Lettuce Wraps 91

Vietnamese Coconut-Lemongrass Chicken... 93

Grilled Chicken and Apple Escarole Salad... 96

Tuscan Chicken Soup with Kale Ribbons... 98

Chicken Larb 100

Chicken Burgers with Szechwan Cashew Sauce 102
Szechwan Cashew Sauce 102
Turkish Chicken Wraps 104
Spanish Cornish Hens.. 106
Pistachio-Roasted Cornish Hens with Arugula, Apricot, and Fennel Salad.............. 108
Duck Breast with Pomegranate and Jicama Salad... 111
Roasted Turkey with Garlicky Mashed Roots... 113
Stuffed Turkey Breast with Pesto Sauce and Arugula Salad.. 115
Spiced Turkey Breast with Cherry BBQ Sauce 117
Wine-Braised Turkey Tenderloin 119
Pan-Sautéed Turkey Breast with Chive Scampi Sauce 122
Braised Turkey Legs with Root Vegetables.. 124
Herbed Turkey Meat Loaf with Caramelized Onion Ketchup and Roasted Cabbage Wedges... 126
Turkey Posole.. 128
Chicken Bone Broth.. 130
Green Harissa Salmon 133
Salmon 133
Harissa... 133
Spiced Sunflower Seeds... 133
Salad 133
Grilled Salmon with Marinated Artichoke Heart Salad 136
Flash-Roasted Chile-Sage Salmon with Green Tomato Salsa 138
Salmon 138
Green Tomato Salsa... 138
Roasted Salmon and Asparagus en Papillote with Lemon-Hazelnut Pesto 140
Spice-Rubbed Salmon with Mushroom-Apple Pan Sauce 142
Sole en Papillote with Julienne Vegetables... 145
Arugula Pesto Fish Tacos with Smoky Lime Cream 147
Almond-Crusted Sole... 149
Grilled Cod and Zucchini Packets with Spicy Mango-Basil Sauce............................. 151
Riesling-Poached Cod with Pesto-Stuffed Tomatoes 153
Broiled Pistachio-Cilantro-Crusted Cod over Smashed Sweet Potatoes................... 155
Rosemary-and-Tangerine Cod with Roasted Broccoli 157
Curried Cod Lettuce Wraps with Pickled Radishes... 159

Roasted Haddock with Lemon and Fennel 161
Pecan-Crusted Snapper with Remoulade and Cajun-Style Okra and Tomatoes 163
Tarragon Tuna Patties with Avocado-Lemon Aïoli 165
Striped Bass Tagine 168
Halibut in Garlic-Shrimp Sauce with Soffrito Collard Greens 170
Seafood Bouillabaisse 172
Classic Shrimp Ceviche 174
Coconut-Crusted Shrimp and Spinach Salad 177
Tropical Shrimp and Scallop Ceviche 179
Jamaican Jerk Shrimp with Avocado Oil 181
Shrimp Scampi with Wilted Spinach and Radicchio 182
Crab Salad with Avocado, Grapefruit, and Jicama 184
Cajun Lobster Tail Boil with Tarragon Aïoli 186
Mussels Frites with Saffron Aïoli 188
Parsnip Frites 188
Saffron Aïoli 188
Mussels 188
Seared Scallops with Beet Relish 191
Grilled Scallops with Cucumber-Dill Salsa 193
Seared Scallops with Tomato, Olive Oil, and Herb Sauce 195
Scallops and Sauce 195
Salad 195
Cumin-Roasted Cauliflower with Fennel and Pearl Onions 197
Chunky Tomato-Eggplant Sauce with Spaghetti Squash 199
Stuffed Portobello Mushrooms 201
Roasted Radicchio 203
Roasted Fennel with Orange Vinaigrette 204
Punjabi-Style Savoy Cabbage 207
Cinnamon-Roasted Butternut Squash 209
Broiled Asparagus with Sieved Egg and Pecans 210
Crunchy Cabbage Slaw with Radishes, Mango, and Mint 212
Roasted Cabbage Rounds with Caraway and Lemon 213
Roasted Cabbage with Orange-Balsamic Drizzle 214
Braised Cabbage with Creamy Dill Sauce and Toasted Walnuts 215
Sautéed Green Cabbage with Toasted Sesame Seeds 216

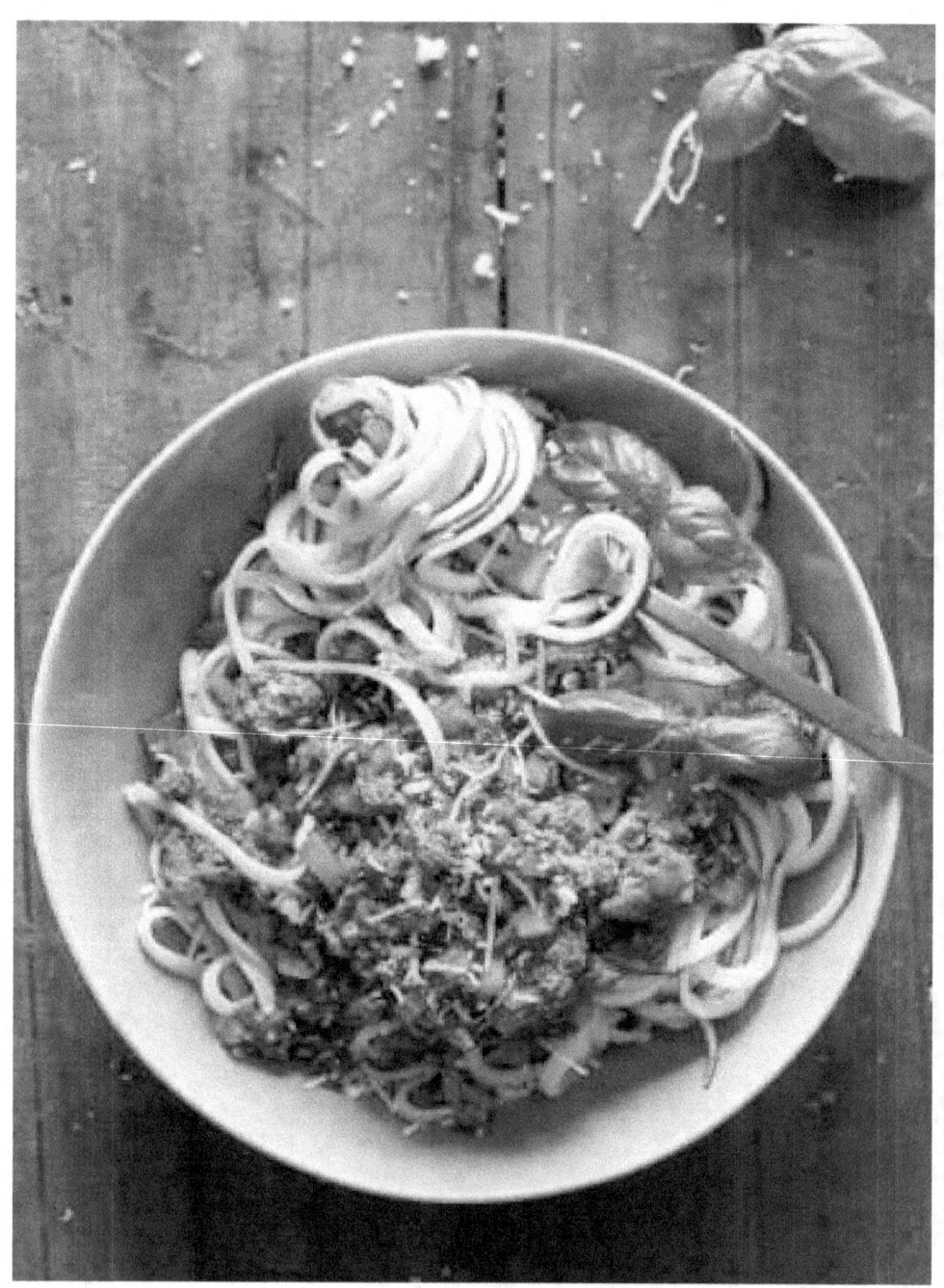

SMOKED BABY BACK RIBS WITH APPLE-MUSTARD MOP SAUCE

SOAK: 1 hour STAND: 15 minutes SMOKE: 4 hours COOK: 20 minutes MAKES: 4 servings
PHOTO

THE RICH FLAVOR AND MEATY TEXTURE OF SMOKED RIBS CALLS FOR SOMETHING COOL AND CRISP TO GO ALONG WITH IT. ALMOST ANY SLAW WILL DO, BUT THE FENNEL SLAW (SEE RECIPE AND PICTURED HERE), IS ESPECIALLY GOOD.

RIBS
- 8 to 10 apple or hickory wood chunks
- 3 to 3½ pounds pork loin baby back ribs
- ¼ cup Smoky Seasoning (see recipe)

SAUCE
- 1 medium cooking apple, peeled, cored, and thinly sliced
- ¼ cup chopped onion
- ¼ cup water
- ¼ cup cider vinegar
- 2 tablespoons Dijon-Style Mustard (see recipe)
- 2 to 3 tablespoons water

1. At least 1 hour before smoke-cooking, soak wood chunks in enough water to cover. Drain before using. Trim visible fat from ribs. If necessary, peel off the thin membrane from the back of the ribs. Place ribs in a large shallow pan. Sprinkle evenly with Smoky Seasoning; rub in with your fingers. Let stand at room temperature for 15 minutes.

2. In a smoker arrange preheated coals, drained wood chunks, and water pan according to the manufacturer's directions. Pour water into pan. Place ribs, bone sides down, on grill rack over water pan. (Or place ribs in a rib rack; place rib

rack on grill rack.) Cover and smoke for 2 hours. Maintain a temperature of about 225°F in the smoker for the duration of smoking. Add additional coals and water as needed to maintain temperature and moisture.

3. Meanwhile, for mop sauce, in a small saucepan combine apple slices, onion, and the ¼ cup water. Bring to boiling; reduce heat. Simmer, covered, for 10 to 12 minutes or until apple slices are very tender, stirring occasionally. Cool slightly; transfer undrained apple and onion to a food processor or blender. Cover and process or blend until smooth. Return puree to saucepan. Stir in vinegar and Dijon-Style Mustard. Cook over medium-low heat for 5 minutes, stirring occasionally. Add 2 to 3 tablespoons of water (or more, as needed) to make the sauce the consistency of a vinaigrette. Divide the sauce into thirds.

4. After 2 hours, brush ribs generously with one-third of the mop sauce. Cover and smoke 1 hour more. Brush again with another one-third of the mop sauce. Wrap each slab of ribs in heavy foil and place the ribs back on the smoker, layering them on top of each other if needed. Cover and smoke for 1 to 1½ hours more or until ribs are tender.*

5. Unwrap ribs and brush with the remaining one-third of the mop sauce. Cut ribs between bones to serve.

*Tip: To test tenderness of the ribs, carefully remove the foil from one of the slabs of ribs. Pick up the rib slab with tongs, holding the slab by the top one-fourth of the slab. Turn the rib slab over so the meaty side is facing down. If the ribs are tender, the slab should begin to fall apart as you pick it up. If it is not tender, wrap again in foil and continue to smoke ribs until tender.

OVEN BBQ COUNTRY-STYLE PORK RIBS WITH FRESH PINEAPPLE SLAW

PREP: 20 minutes COOK: 8 minutes BAKE: 1 hour 15 minutes MAKES: 4 servings

COUNTRY-STYLE PORK RIBS ARE MEATY, INEXPENSIVE, AND, IF TREATED THE RIGHT WAY—SUCH AS COOKED LOW AND SLOW IN A MESS OF BARBECUE SAUCE—GET MELTINGLY TENDER.

2 pounds boneless country-style pork ribs
¼ teaspoon black pepper
1 tablespoon refined coconut oil
½ cup fresh orange juice
1½ cups BBQ Sauce (see recipe)
3 cups shredded green and/or red cabbage
1 cup shredded carrots
2 cups finely chopped pineapple
⅓ cup Bright Citrus Vinaigrette (see recipe)
BBQ Sauce (see recipe) (optional)

1. Preheat oven to 350°F. Sprinkle pork with pepper. In an extra-large skillet heat coconut oil over medium-high heat. Add pork ribs; cook for 8 to 10 minutes or until browned, turning to brown evenly. Place ribs in a 3-quart rectangular baking dish.

2. For sauce, add orange juice to skillet, stirring to scrape up any browned bits. Stir in the 1½ cups BBQ Sauce. Pour sauce over ribs. Turn ribs to coat with sauce (if necessary, use a pastry brush to brush sauce over ribs). Cover baking dish tightly with aluminum foil.

3. Bake ribs for 1 hour. Remove foil and brush ribs with sauce from baking dish. Bake about 15 minutes more or until

ribs are tender and browned and sauce has thickened slightly.

4. Meanwhile, for pineapple slaw, combine cabbage, carrots, pineapple, and Bright Citrus Vinaigrette. Cover and refrigerate until serving time.

5. Serve ribs with slaw and, if desired, additional BBQ Sauce.

SPICY PORK GOULASH

PREP: 20 minutes COOK: 40 minutes MAKES: 6 servings

THIS HUNGARIAN-STYLE STEW IS SERVED ON A BED OF CRUNCHY, BARELY WILTED CABBAGE FOR A ONE-DISH MEAL. CRUSH THE CARAWAY SEEDS IN A MORTAR AND PESTLE IF YOU HAVE ONE. IF NOT, CRUSH THEM UNDER THE BROAD SIDE OF A CHEF'S KNIFE BY PRESSING DOWN ON KNIFE GENTLY WITH YOUR FIST.

GOULASH

- 1½ pounds ground pork
- 2 cups chopped red, orange, and/or yellow sweet peppers
- ¾ cup finely chopped red onion
- 1 small fresh red chile, seeded and finely chopped (see tip)
- 4 teaspoons Smoky Seasoning (see recipe)
- 1 teaspoon caraway seeds, crushed
- ¼ teaspoon ground marjoram or oregano
- 1 14-ounce can no-salt-added diced tomatoes, undrained
- 2 tablespoons red wine vinegar
- 1 tablespoon finely shredded lemon peel
- ⅓ cup snipped fresh parsley

CABBAGE

- 2 tablespoons olive oil
- 1 medium onion, sliced
- 1 small head green or red cabbage, cored and thinly sliced

1. For the goulash, in a large Dutch oven cook ground pork, sweet peppers, and onion over medium-high heat for 8 to 10 minutes or until the pork is no longer pink and vegetables are crisp-tender, stirring with a wooden spoon to break up meat. Drain off fat. Reduce heat to low; add

red chile, Smoky Seasoning, caraway seeds, and marjoram. Cover and cook for 10 minutes. Add undrained tomatoes and vinegar. Bring to boiling; reduce heat. Simmer, covered, for 20 minutes.

2. Meanwhile, for cabbage, in an extra-large skillet heat oil over medium heat. Add onion and cook until softened, about 2 minutes. Add cabbage; stir to combine. Reduce heat to low. Cook about 8 minutes or until cabbage is just tender, stirring occasionally.

3. To serve, place some of the cabbage mixture on a plate. Top with goulash and sprinkle with lemon zest and parsley.

ITALIAN SAUSAGE MEATBALLS MARINARA WITH SLICED FENNEL AND ONION SAUTÉ

PREP: 30 minutes BAKE: 30 minutes COOK: 40 minutes MAKES: 4 to 6 servings

THIS RECIPE IS A RARE EXAMPLE OF A CANNED PRODUCT WORKING AS WELL AS—IF NOT BETTER THAN—THE FRESH VERSION. UNLESS YOU HAVE TOMATOES THAT ARE VERY, VERY RIPE, YOU WILL NOT GET AS GOOD A CONSISTENCY IN A SAUCE USING FRESH TOMATOES AS YOU CAN USING CANNED TOMATOES. JUST BE SURE YOU USE A NO-SALT-ADDED PRODUCT—AND, EVEN BETTER, ORGANIC.

MEATBALLS
- 2 large eggs
- ½ cup almond meal
- 8 cloves garlic, minced
- 6 tablespoons dry white wine
- 1 tablespoon paprika
- 2 teaspoons black pepper
- 1 teaspoon fennel seeds, lightly crushed
- 1 teaspoon dried oregano, crushed
- 1 teaspoon dried thyme, crushed
- ¼ to ½ teaspoon cayenne pepper
- 1½ pounds ground pork

MARINARA
- 2 tablespoons olive oil
- 2 15-ounce cans no-salt-added crushed tomatoes or one 28-ounce can no-salt-added crushed tomatoes
- ½ cup snipped fresh basil
- 3 medium fennel bulbs, halved, cored, and thinly sliced

1 large sweet onion, halved and thinly sliced

1. Preheat oven to 375°F. Line a large rimmed baking sheet with parchment paper; set aside. In a large bowl whisk together the eggs, almond meal, 6 cloves of the minced garlic, 3 tablespoons of the wine, the paprika, 1½ teaspoons of the black pepper, the fennel seeds, oregano, thyme, and cayenne pepper. Add the pork; mix well. Shape pork mixture into 1½-inch meatballs (should have about 24 meatballs); arrange in a single layer on the prepared baking sheet. Bake about 30 minutes or until lightly browned, turning once while baking.

2. Meanwhile, for marinara sauce, in a 4- to 6-quart Dutch oven heat 1 tablespoon of the olive oil. Add the 2 remaining cloves minced garlic; cook about 1 minute or until just starting to brown. Quickly add the remaining 3 tablespoons wine, the crushed tomatoes, and the basil. Bring to boiling; reduce heat. Simmer, uncovered, for 5 minutes. Carefully stir the cooked meatballs into the marinara sauce. Cover and simmer for 25 to 30 minutes.

3. Meanwhile, in a large skillet heat the remaining 1 tablespoon olive oil over medium heat. Stir in the sliced fennel and onion. Cook for 8 to 10 minutes or until just tender and lightly browned, stirring frequently. Season with the remaining ½ teaspoon black pepper. Serve the meatballs and marinara sauce over the fennel and onion sauté.

PORK-STUFFED ZUCCHINI BOATS WITH BASIL AND PINE NUTS

PREP: 20 minutes COOK: 22 minutes BAKE: 20 minutes MAKES: 4 servings

KIDS WILL LOVE THIS FUN-TO-EAT DISH OF HOLLOWED-OUT ZUCCHINI STUFFED WITH GROUND PORK, TOMATOES, AND SWEET PEPPERS. IF YOU LIKE, STIR IN 3 TABLESPOONS OF BASIL PESTO (SEE RECIPE) IN PLACE OF THE FRESH BASIL, PARSLEY, AND PINE NUTS.

- 2 medium zucchini
- 1 tablespoon extra virgin olive oil
- 12 ounces ground pork
- ¾ cup chopped onion
- 2 cloves garlic, minced
- 1 cup chopped tomatoes
- ⅔ cup finely chopped yellow or orange sweet pepper
- 1 teaspoon fennel seeds, lightly crushed
- ½ teaspoon crushed red pepper flakes
- ¼ cup snipped fresh basil
- 3 tablespoons snipped fresh parsley
- 2 tablespoons pine nuts, toasted (see tip) and coarsely chopped
- 1 teaspoon finely shredded lemon peel

1. Preheat oven to 350°F. Halve zucchini lengthwise and carefully scrape out the center, leaving ¼-inch-thick shell. Coarsely chop the zucchini pulp and set aside. Arrange zucchini halves, cut sides up, on a foil-lined baking sheet.

2. For filling, in a large skillet heat the olive oil over medium-high heat. Add ground pork; cook until no longer pink, stirring with a wooden spoon to break up meat. Drain off fat. Reduce heat to medium. Add the reserved zucchini

pulp, onion, and garlic; cook and stir about 8 minutes or until onion is soft. Stir in the tomatoes, sweet pepper, fennel seeds, and crushed red pepper. Cook about 10 minutes or until tomatoes are soft and beginning to break down. Remove pan from heat. Stir in the basil, parsley, pine nuts, and lemon peel. Divide filling among zucchini shells, mounding slightly. Bake for 20 to 25 minutes or until zucchini shells are crisp-tender.

CURRIED PORK AND PINEAPPLE "NOODLE" BOWLS WITH COCONUT MILK AND HERBS

PREP: 30 minutes COOK: 15 minutes BAKE: 40 minutes MAKES: 4 servings PHOTO

1 large spaghetti squash

2 tablespoons refined coconut oil

1 pound ground pork

2 tablespoons finely chopped scallions

2 tablespoons fresh lime juice

1 tablespoon minced fresh ginger

6 cloves garlic, minced

1 tablespoon minced lemongrass

1 tablespoon no-salt-added Thai-style red curry powder

1 cup chopped red sweet pepper

1 cup chopped onion

½ cup julienne-cut carrot

1 baby bok choy, sliced (3 cups)

1 cup sliced fresh button mushrooms

1 or 2 Thai bird chiles, thinly sliced (see tip)

1 13.5-ounce can natural coconut milk (such as Nature's Way)

½ cup Chicken Bone Broth (see recipe) or no-salt-added chicken broth

¼ cup fresh pineapple juice

3 tablespoons unsalted no-oil-added cashew butter

1 cup cubed fresh pineapple, cubed

Lime wedges

Fresh cilantro, mint, and/or Thai basil

Chopped roasted cashews

1. Preheat oven to 400°F. Microwave spaghetti squash on high for 3 minutes. Carefully cut the squash in half lengthwise

and scrape out the seeds. Rub 1 tablespoon of the coconut oil over the cut sides of the squash. Place squash halves, cut sides down, on a baking sheet. Bake for 40 to 50 minutes or until squash can be pierced easily with a knife. Using the tines of a fork, scrape the flesh from the shells and keep warm until ready to serve.

2. Meanwhile, in a medium bowl combine the pork, scallions, lime juice, ginger, garlic, lemongrass, and curry powder; mix well. In an extra-large skillet heat the remaining 1 tablespoon of the coconut oil over medium-high heat. Add pork mixture; cook until no longer pink, stirring with a wooden spoon to break up meat. Add the sweet pepper, onion, and carrot; cook and stir about 3 minutes or until vegetables are crisp-tender. Stir in the bok choy, mushrooms, chiles, coconut milk, Chicken Bone Broth, pineapple juice, and cashew butter. Bring to boiling; reduce heat. Add pineapple; simmer, uncovered, until heated through.

3. To serve, divide the spaghetti squash among four serving bowls. Ladle the curried pork over the squash. Serve with lime wedges, herbs, and cashews.

SPICY GRILLED PORK PATTIES WITH TANGY CUCUMBER SALAD

PREP: 30 minutes GRILL: 10 minutes STAND: 10 minutes MAKES: 4 servings

THE CRUNCHY CUCUMBER SALAD FLAVORED WITH FRESH MINT IS A COOLING AND REFRESHING COMPLEMENT TO THE SPICY PORK BURGERS.

- ⅓ cup olive oil
- ¼ cup chopped fresh mint
- 3 tablespoons white wine vinegar
- 8 cloves garlic, minced
- ¼ teaspoon black pepper
- 2 medium cucumbers, very thinly sliced
- 1 small onion, cut into thin slivers (about ½ cup)
- 1¼ to 1½ pounds ground pork
- ¼ cup chopped fresh cilantro
- 1 to 2 medium fresh jalapeño or serrano chile peppers, seeded (if desired) and finely chopped (see tip)
- 2 medium red sweet peppers, seeded and quartered
- 2 teaspoons olive oil

1. In a large bowl whisk together ⅓ cup olive oil, mint, vinegar, 2 cloves minced garlic, and the black pepper. Add sliced cucumbers and onion. Toss until well coated. Cover and chill until ready to serve, stirring once or twice.

2. In a large bowl combine pork, cilantro, chile pepper, and the remaining 6 cloves minced garlic. Shape into four ¾-inch-thick patties. Brush pepper quarters lightly with the 2 teaspoons olive oil.

3. For a charcoal or gas grill, place patties and sweet pepper quarters directly over medium heat. Cover and grill until an instant-read thermometer inserted into sides of pork patties registers 160°F and pepper quarters are tender and lightly charred, turning patties and pepper quarters once halfway through grilling. Allow 10 to 12 minutes for patties and 8 to 10 minutes for the pepper quarters.

4. When pepper quarters are done, wrap them in a piece of foil to completely enclose. Let stand about 10 minutes or until cool enough to handle. Using a sharp knife, carefully peel off the pepper skins. Thinly slice pepper quarters lengthwise.

5. To serve, stir cucumber salad and spoon evenly onto four large serving plates. Add a pork patty to each plate. Pile the red pepper slices evenly on top of patties.

ZUCCHINI-CRUST PIZZA WITH SUN-DRIED TOMATO PESTO, SWEET PEPPERS, AND ITALIAN SAUSAGE

PREP: 30 minutes COOK: 15 minutes BAKE: 30 minutes MAKES: 4 servings

THIS IS KNIFE-AND-FORK PIZZA. BE SURE TO PRESS THE SAUSAGE AND PEPPERS LIGHTLY INTO THE PESTO-COATED CRUST SO THAT THE TOPPINGS ADHERE ENOUGH FOR THE PIZZA TO CUT NEATLY.

2 tablespoons olive oil
1 tablespoon finely ground almonds
1 large egg, lightly beaten
½ cup almond flour
1 tablespoon snipped fresh oregano
¼ teaspoon black pepper
3 cloves garlic, minced
3½ cups shredded zucchini (2 medium)
Italian Sausage (see recipe, below)
1 tablespoon extra virgin olive oil
1 sweet pepper (yellow, red, or half of each), seeded and cut into very thin strips
1 small onion, thinly sliced
Sun-Dried Tomato Pesto (see recipe, below)

1. Preheat oven to 425°F. Brush a 12-inch pizza pan with the 2 tablespoons olive oil. Sprinkle with ground almonds; set aside.

2. For crust, in a large bowl combine egg, almond flour, oregano, black pepper, and garlic. Place shredded zucchini in a clean towel or piece of cheesecloth. Wrap tightly

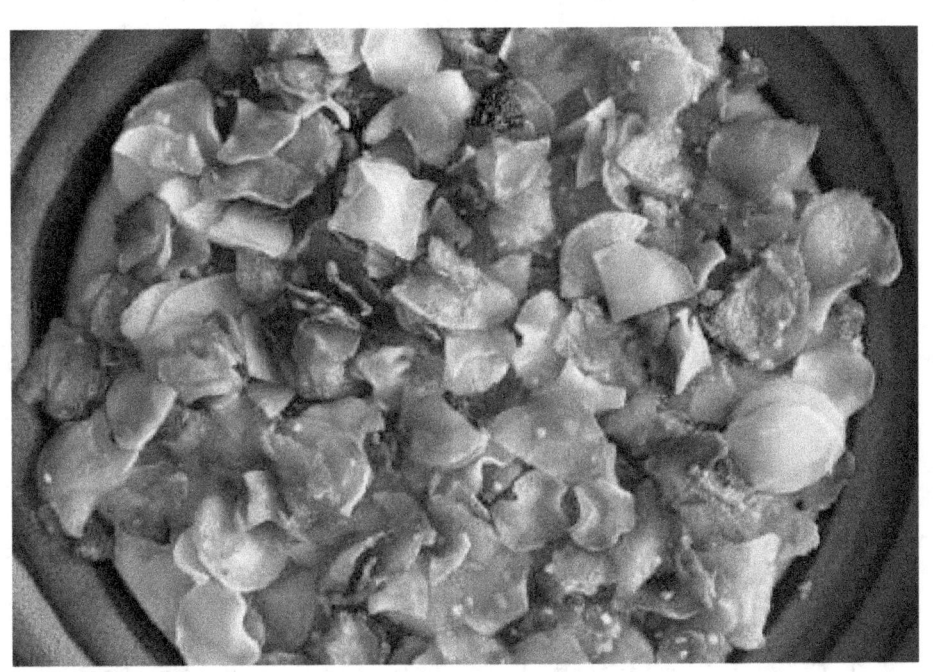

SMOKED LEMON-CORIANDER LAMB LEG WITH GRILLED ASPARAGUS

SOAK: 30 minutes PREP: 20 minutes GRILL: 45 minutes STAND: 10 minutes MAKES: 6 to 8 servings

SIMPLE BUT ELEGANT, THIS DISH FEATURES TWO INGREDIENTS THAT COME INTO THEIR OWN IN THE SPRING—LAMB AND ASPARAGUS. TOASTING THE CORIANDER SEEDS ENHANCES THE WARM, EARTHY, SLIGHTLY TANGY FLAVOR.

1 cup hickory wood chips

2 tablespoons coriander seeds

2 tablespoons finely shredded lemon peel

1½ teaspoons black pepper

2 tablespoons snipped fresh thyme

1 2- to 3-pound boneless leg of lamb

2 bunches fresh asparagus

1 tablespoon olive oil

¼ teaspoon black pepper

1 lemon, cut into quarters

1. At least 30 minutes before smoke-cooking, in a bowl soak hickory chips in enough water to cover; set aside. Meanwhile, in a small skillet toast coriander seeds over medium heat about 2 minutes or until fragrant and crackling, stirring frequently. Remove seeds from skillet; let cool. When seeds have cooled, coarsely crush in a mortar and pestle (or place seeds on a cutting board and crush them with the back of a wooden spoon). In a small bowl combine crushed coriander seeds, lemon peel, the 1½ teaspoons pepper, and thyme; set aside.

2. Remove netting from lamb roast if present. On a work surface open up the roast, fat side down. Sprinkle half of the spice mixture over meat; rub in with your fingers. Roll the roast up and tie with four to six pieces of 100%-cotton kitchen string. Sprinkle the remaining spice mixture over outside of roast, pressing lightly to adhere.

3. For a charcoal grill, arrange medium-hot coals around a drip pan. Test for medium heat above the pan. Sprinkle the drained wood chips over the coals. Place lamb roast on the grill rack over the drip pan. Cover and smoke for 40 to 50 minutes for medium (145°F). (For a gas grill, preheat grill. Reduce heat to medium. Adjust for indirect cooking. Smoke as above, except add drained wood chips according to manufacturer's directions.) Cover roast loosely with foil. Let stand for 10 minutes before slicing.

4. Meanwhile, trim woody ends from asparagus. In a large bowl toss asparagus with olive oil and the ¼ teaspoon pepper. Place asparagus around outer edges of grill, directly over the coals and perpendicular to the grill grate. Cover and grill for 5 to 6 minutes until crisp-tender. Squeeze lemon wedges over asparagus.

5. Remove string from lamb roast and thinly slice meat. Serve meat with grilled asparagus.

LAMB HOT POT

PREP: 30 minutes COOK: 2 hours 40 minutes MAKES: 4 servings

WARM UP WITH THIS SAVORY STEW ON A FALL OR WINTER NIGHT. THE STEW IS SERVED OVER A VELVETY CELERY ROOT-PARSNIP MASH FLAVORED WITH DIJON-STYLE MUSTARD, CASHEW CREAM, AND CHIVES. NOTE: CELERY ROOT IS SOMETIMES CALLED CELERIAC.

- 10 black peppercorns
- 6 sage leaves
- 3 whole allspice
- 2 2-inch strips orange peel
- 2 pounds boneless lamb shoulder
- 3 tablespoons olive oil
- 2 medium onions, coarsely chopped
- 1 14.5-ounce can no-salt-added diced tomatoes, undrained
- 1½ cups Beef Bone Broth (see recipe) or no-salt-added beef broth
- ¾ cup dry white wine
- 3 large cloves garlic, crushed and peeled
- 2 pounds celery root, peeled and cut into 1-inch cubes
- 6 medium parsnips, peeled and cut into 1-inch slices (about 2 pounds)
- 2 tablespoons olive oil
- 2 tablespoons Cashew Cream (see recipe)
- 1 tablespoon Dijon-Style Mustard (see recipe)
- ¼ cup snipped chives

1. For the bouquet garni, cut a 7-inch square of cheesecloth. Place peppercorns, sage, allspice, and orange peel in center of cheesecloth. Bring up the corners of the cheesecloth and tie securely with clean 100%-cotton kitchen string. Set aside.

2. Trim fat from lamb shoulder; cut lamb into 1-inch pieces. In a Dutch oven heat the 3 tablespoons olive oil over medium heat. Cook lamb, in batches if necessary, in hot oil until browned; remove from pan and keep warm. Add onions to pan; cook for 5 to 8 minutes or until softened and lightly browned. Add bouquet garni, undrained tomatoes, 1¼ cups of the Beef Bone Broth, wine, and garlic. Bring to boiling; reduce heat. Simmer, covered, for 2 hours, stirring occasionally. Remove and discard bouquet garni.

3. Meanwhile, for mash, place celery root and parsnips in a large stockpot; cover with water. Bring to boiling over medium-high heat; reduce heat to low. Cover and simmer gently for 30 to 40 minutes or until the vegetables are very tender when pierced with a fork. Drain; place vegetables in a food processor. Add the remaining ¼ cup Beef Bone Broth and the 2 tablespoons oil; pulse until mash is almost smooth but still has some texture, stopping once or twice to scrape down the sides. Transfer mash to a bowl. Stir in Cashew Cream, mustard, and chives.

4. To serve, divide mash among four bowls; top with Lamb Hot Pot.

LAMB STEW WITH CELERY-ROOT NOODLES

PREP: 30 minutes BAKE: 1 hour 30 minutes MAKES: 6 servings

CELERY ROOT TAKES AN ENTIRELY DIFFERENT FORM IN THIS STEW THAN IT DOES IN THE LAMB HOT POT (SEE <u>RECIPE</u>). A MANDOLINE SLICER IS USED TO CREATE VERY THIN STRIPS OF THE SWEET AND NUTTY-TASTING ROOT. THE "NOODLES" SIMMER IN THE STEW UNTIL THEY ARE TENDER.

- 2 teaspoons Lemon-Herb Seasoning (see <u>recipe</u>)
- 1½ pounds lamb stew meat, cut into 1-inch cubes
- 2 tablespoons olive oil
- 2 cups chopped onions
- 1 cup chopped carrots
- 1 cup diced turnips
- 1 tablespoon minced garlic (6 cloves)
- 2 tablespoons no-salt-added tomato paste
- ½ cup dry red wine
- 4 cups Beef Bone Broth (see <u>recipe</u>) or no-salt-added beef broth
- 1 bay leaf
- 2 cups 1-inch cubes butternut squash
- 1 cup diced eggplant
- 1 pound celery root, peeled
- Chopped fresh parsley

1. Preheat oven to 250°F. Sprinkle Lemon-Herb Seasoning evenly over lamb. Toss gently to coat. Heat a 6- to 8-quart Dutch oven over medium-high heat. Add 1 tablespoon of the olive oil and half of the seasoned lamb to the Dutch oven. Brown meat in hot oil on all sides; transfer browned

meat to a plate and repeat with remaining lamb and olive oil. Reduce heat to medium.

2. Add onions, carrots, and turnips to pot. Cook and stir vegetables for 4 minutes; add garlic and tomato paste and cook 1 minute more. Add red wine, Beef Bone Broth, bay leaf, and reserved meat and any accumulated juices to pot. Bring mixture to a simmer. Cover and place Dutch oven in preheated oven. Bake for 1 hour. Stir in butternut squash and eggplant. Return to oven and bake for an additional 30 minutes.

3. While stew is in oven, use a mandoline to very thinly slice celery root. Cut celery root slices into ½-inch-wide strips. (You should have about 4 cups.) Stir celery root strips into stew. Simmer about 10 minutes or until tender. Remove and discard bay leaf before serving stew. Sprinkle each serving with chopped parsley.

FRENCHED LAMB CHOPS WITH POMEGRANATE-DATE CHUTNEY

PREP: 10 minutes COOK: 18 minutes COOL: 10 minutes MAKES: 4 servings

THE TERM "FRENCHED" REFERS TO A RIB BONE FROM WHICH FAT, MEAT, AND CONNECTIVE TISSUE HAVE BEEN REMOVED WITH A SHARP PARING KNIFE. IT MAKES FOR AN ATTRACTIVE PRESENTATION. ASK YOUR BUTCHER TO DO IT OR YOU CAN DO IT YOURSELF.

CHUTNEY
½ cup unsweetened pomegranate juice
1 tablespoon fresh lemon juice
1 shallot, peeled and thinly sliced into rings
1 teaspoon finely shredded orange peel
⅓ cup chopped Medjool dates
¼ teaspoon crushed red pepper
¼ cup pomegranate arils*
1 tablespoon olive oil
1 tablespoon chopped fresh Italian (flat-leaf) parsley

LAMB CHOPS
2 tablespoons olive oil
8 frenched lamb rib chops

1. For the chutney, in a small skillet combine pomegranate juice, lemon juice, and shallot. Bring to boiling; reduce heat. Simmer, uncovered, for 2 minutes. Add orange peel, dates, and crushed red pepper. Let stand until cool, about 10 minutes. Stir in pomegranate arils, the 1 tablespoon olive oil, and the parsley. Set aside at room temperature until serving time.

2. For the chops, in a large skillet heat the 2 tablespoons olive oil over medium heat. Working in batches, add chops to skillet and cook for 6 to 8 minutes for medium rare (145°F), turning once. Top chops with chutney.

*Note: Fresh pomegranates and their arils, or seeds, are available from October through February. If you can't find them, use unsweetened dried seeds to add crunch to the chutney.

CHIMICHURRI LAMB LOIN CHOPS WITH SAUTÉED RADICCHIO SLAW

PREP: 30 minutes MARINATE: 20 minutes COOK: 20 minutes MAKES: 4 servings

IN ARGENTINA, CHIMICHURRI IS THE MOST POPULAR CONDIMENT ACCOMPANYING THAT COUNTRY'S RENOWNED GAUCHO-STYLE GRILLED STEAK. THERE ARE LOTS OF VARIATIONS, BUT THE THICK HERB SAUCE IS USUALLY BUILT AROUND PARSLEY, CILANTRO OR OREGANO, SHALLOTS AND/OR GARLIC, CRUSHED RED PEPPER, OLIVE OIL, AND RED WINE VINEGAR. IT'S GREAT ON GRILLED STEAK BUT EQUALLY BRILLIANT ON ROASTED OR PAN-SEARED LAMB CHOPS, CHICKEN, AND PORK.

8 lamb loin chops, cut 1 inch thick
½ cup Chimichurri Sauce (see recipe)
2 tablespoons olive oil
1 sweet onion, halved and sliced
1 teaspoon cumin seeds, crushed*
1 clove garlic, minced
1 head radicchio, cored and sliced into thin ribbons
1 tablespoon balsamic vinegar

1. Place lamb chops in an extra-large bowl. Drizzle with 2 tablespoons of the Chimichurri Sauce. Using your fingers, rub the sauce over the entire surface of each chop. Let chops marinate at room temperature for 20 minutes.

2. Meanwhile, for sautéed radicchio slaw, in an extra-large skillet heat 1 tablespoon of the olive oil. Add onion, cumin seeds, and garlic; cook for 6 to 7 minutes or until onion softens, stirring frequently. Add radicchio; cook for 1 to 2

minutes or until radicchio just wilts slightly. Transfer slaw to a large bowl. Add balsamic vinegar and toss well to combine. Cover and keep warm.

3. Wipe out skillet. Add the remaining 1 tablespoon olive oil to the skillet and heat over medium-high heat. Add the lamb chops; reduce heat to medium. Cook for 9 to 11 minutes or until desired doneness, turning chops occasionally with tongs.

4. Serve chops with slaw and the remaining Chimichurri Sauce.

*Note: To crush cumin seeds, use a mortar and pestle—or place seeds on a cutting board and crush with a chef's knife.

ANCHO-AND-SAGE-RUBBED LAMB CHOPS WITH CARROT-SWEET POTATO REMOULADE

PREP: 12 minutes CHILL: 1 to 2 hours GRILL: 6 minutes MAKES: 4 servings

THERE ARE THREE TYPES OF LAMB CHOPS. THICK AND MEATY LOIN CHOPS LOOK LIKE SMALL T-BONE STEAKS. RIB CHOPS—CALLED FOR HERE—ARE CREATED BY CUTTING BETWEEN THE BONES OF A RACK OF LAMB. THEY ARE VERY TENDER AND HAVE A LONG, ATTRACTIVE BONE ON THE SIDE. THEY ARE OFTEN SERVED PAN-SEARED OR GRILLED. BUDGET-FRIENDLY SHOULDER CHOPS ARE A BIT FATTIER AND LESS TENDER THAN THE OTHER TWO TYPES. THEY ARE BEST BROWNED AND THEN BRAISED IN WINE, STOCK, AND TOMATOES—OR SOME COMBINATION OF THEM.

- 3 medium carrots, coarsely shredded
- 2 small sweet potatoes, julienne-cut* or coarsely shredded
- ½ cup Paleo Mayo (see recipe)
- 2 tablespoons fresh lemon juice
- 2 teaspoons Dijon-Style Mustard (see recipe)
- 2 tablespoons snipped fresh parsley
- ½ teaspoon black pepper
- 8 lamb rib chops, cut ½ to ¾ inch thick
- 2 tablespoon snipped fresh sage or 2 teaspoons dried sage, crushed
- 2 teaspoons ground ancho chile pepper
- ½ teaspoon garlic powder

1. For the remoulade, in a medium bowl combine carrots and sweet potatoes. In a small bowl stir together Paleo Mayo, lemon juice, Dijon-Style Mustard, parsley, and black

pepper. Pour over carrots and sweet potatoes; toss to coat. Cover and chill for 1 to 2 hours.

2. Meanwhile, in a small bowl combine sage, ancho chile, and garlic powder. Rub spice mixture onto lamb chops.

3. For a charcoal or gas grill, place lamb chops on a grill rack directly over medium heat. Cover and grill for 6 to 8 minutes for medium rare (145°F) or 10 to 12 minutes for medium (150°F), turning once halfway through grilling.

4. Serve the lamb chops with the remoulade.

*Note: Use a mandoline with a julienne attachment to cut the sweet potatoes.

LAMB CHOPS WITH SHALLOT, MINT, AND OREGANO RUB

PREP: 20 minutes MARINATE: 1 to 24 hours ROAST: 40 minutes GRILL: 12 minutes
MAKES: 4 servings

AS WITH MOST MARINATED MEATS, THE LONGER YOU LEAVE THE HERB RUB ON THE LAMB CHOPS BEFORE COOKING, THE MORE FLAVORFUL THEY WILL BE. THERE IS AN EXCEPTION TO THIS RULE, AND THAT IS WHEN YOU ARE USING A MARINADE THAT CONTAINS HIGHLY ACIDIC INGREDIENTS SUCH AS CITRUS JUICE, VINEGAR, AND WINE. IF YOU LET THE MEAT SIT IN AN ACIDIC MARINADE TOO LONG, IT BEGINS TO BREAK DOWN AND GET MUSHY.

LAMB
- 2 tablespoons finely chopped shallot
- 2 tablespoons finely chopped fresh mint
- 2 tablespoons finely chopped fresh oregano
- 5 teaspoons Mediterranean Seasoning (see recipe)
- 4 teaspoons olive oil
- 2 cloves garlic, minced
- 8 lamb rib chops, cut about 1 inch thick

SALAD
- ¾ pound baby beets, trimmed
- 1 tablespoon olive oil
- ¼ cup fresh lemon juice
- ¼ cup olive oil
- 1 tablespoon finely chopped shallot
- 1 teaspoon Dijon-Style Mustard (see recipe)
- 6 cups mixed greens
- 4 teaspoons snipped chives

1. For the lamb, in a small bowl combine 2 tablespoons shallot, mint, oregano, 4 teaspoons of the Mediterranean seasoning, and 4 teaspoons olive oil. Sprinkle rub over all sides of the lamb chops; rub in with your fingers. Place chops on a plate; cover with plastic wrap and refrigerate for at least 1 hour or up to 24 hours to marinate.

2. For salad, preheat oven to 400°F. Scrub beets well; cut into wedges. Place in a 2-quart baking dish. Drizzle with the 1 tablespoon olive oil. Cover dish with foil. Roast about 40 minutes or until beets are tender. Cool completely. (Beets can be roasted up to 2 days ahead.)

3. In a screw-top jar combine lemon juice, ¼ cup olive oil, 1 tablespoon shallot, Dijon-Style Mustard, and the remaining 1 teaspoon Mediterranean Seasoning. Cover and shake well. In a salad bowl combine beets and greens; toss with some of the vinaigrette.

4. For a charcoal or gas grill, place chops on the greased grill rack directly over medium heat. Cover and grill to desired doneness, turning once halfway through grilling. Allow 12 to 14 minutes for medium rare (145°F) or 15 to 17 minutes for medium (160°F).

5. To serve, place 2 lamb chops and some of the salad on each of four serving plates. Sprinkle with chives. Pass remaining vinaigrette.

GARDEN-STUFFED LAMB BURGERS WITH RED PEPPER COULIS

PREP: 20 minutes STAND: 15 minutes GRILL: 27 minutes MAKES: 4 servings

A COULIS IS NOTHING MORE THAN A SIMPLE, SMOOTH SAUCE MADE FROM PUREED FRUITS OR VEGETABLES. THE BRIGHT AND BEAUTIFUL RED PEPPER SAUCE FOR THESE LAMB BURGERS GETS A DOUBLE DOSE OF SMOKE—FROM GRILLING AND FROM A SHOT OF SMOKED PAPRIKA.

RED PEPPER COULIS
- 1 large red sweet pepper
- 1 tablespoon dry white wine or white wine vinegar
- 1 teaspoon olive oil
- ½ teaspoon smoked paprika

BURGERS
- ¼ cup snipped unsulfured dried tomatoes
- ¼ cup shredded zucchini
- 1 tablespoon snipped fresh basil
- 2 teaspoons olive oil
- ½ teaspoon black pepper
- 1½ pounds ground lamb
- 1 egg white, lightly beaten
- 1 tablespoon Mediterranean Seasoning (see recipe)

1. For the red pepper coulis, place the red pepper on the grill rack directly over medium heat. Cover and grill for 15 to 20 minutes or until charred and very tender, turning the pepper about every 5 minutes to char each side. Remove from the grill and immediately place in a paper bag or foil to completely enclose the pepper. Let stand for 15

minutes or until cool enough to handle. Using a sharp knife, gently pull off skins and discard. Quarter pepper lengthwise and remove stems, seeds, and membranes. In a food processor combine the roasted pepper, wine, olive oil, and smoked paprika. Cover and process or blend until smooth.

2. Meanwhile, for the filling, place dried tomatoes in a small bowl and cover with boiling water. Let stand for 5 minutes; drain. Pat tomatoes and shredded zucchini dry with paper towels. In the small bowl stir together tomatoes, zucchini, basil, olive oil, and ¼ teaspoon of the black pepper; set aside.

3. In a large bowl combine ground lamb, egg white, remaining ¼ teaspoon black pepper, and Mediterranean Seasoning; mix well. Divide meat mixture into eight equal portions and shape each into a ¼-inch-thick patty. Spoon filling onto four of the patties; top with remaining patties and pinch edges to seal in the filling.

4. Place patties on the grill rack directly over medium heat. Cover and grill for 12 to 14 minutes or until done (160°F), turning once halfway through grilling.

5. To serve, top burgers with red pepper coulis.

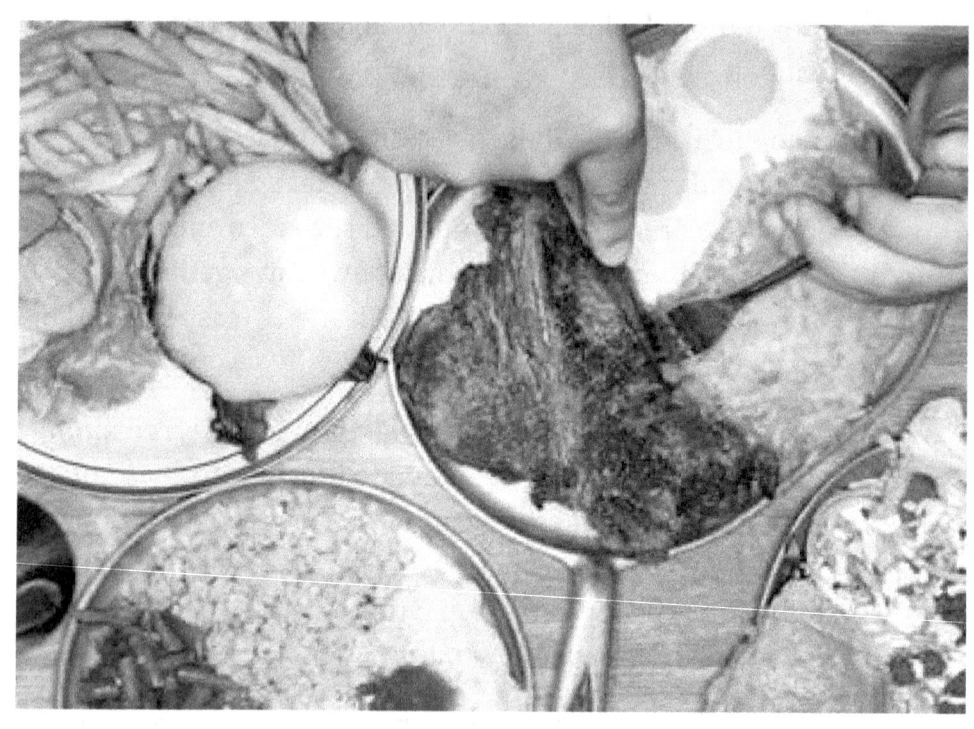

DOUBLE-OREGANO LAMB KABOBS WITH TZATZIKI SAUCE

SOAK: 30 minutes PREP: 20 minutes CHILL: 30 minutes GRILL: 8 minutes MAKES: 4 servings

THESE LAMB KABOBS ARE ESSENTIALLY WHAT IS KNOWN AS KOFTA IN THE MEDITERRANEAN AND MIDDLE EAST—SEASONED GROUND MEAT (USUALLY LAMB OR BEEF) IS SHAPED INTO BALLS OR AROUND A SKEWER AND THEN GRILLED. FRESH AND DRIED OREGANO GIVE THEM GREAT GREEK FLAVOR.

8 10-inch wooden skewers

LAMB KABOBS

1½ pounds lean ground lamb

1 small onion, shredded and squeezed dry

1 tablespoon snipped fresh oregano

2 teaspoon dried oregano, crushed

1 teaspoon black pepper

TZATZIKI SAUCE

1 cup Paleo Mayo (see recipe)

½ of a large cucumber, seeded and shredded and squeezed dry

2 tablespoons fresh lemon juice

1 clove garlic, minced

1. Soak skewers in enough water to cover for 30 minutes.

2. For lamb kabobs, in a large bowl combine ground lamb, onion, fresh and dried oregano, and pepper; mix well. Divide the lamb mixture into eight equal portions. Shape each portion around half of a skewer, creating a 5×1-inch log. Cover and chill for at least 30 minutes.

3. Meanwhile, for Tzatziki Sauce, in a small bowl combine Paleo Mayo, cucumber, lemon juice, and garlic. Cover and chill until serving.

4. For a charcoal or gas grill, place lamb kabobs on grill rack directly over medium heat. Cover and grill about 8 minutes for medium (160°F), turning once halfway through grilling.

5. Serve lamb kabobs with Tzatziki Sauce.

ROAST CHICKEN WITH SAFFRON AND LEMON

PREP: 15 minutes CHILL: 8 hours ROAST: 1 hour 15 minutes STAND: 10 minutes MAKES: 4 servings

SAFFRON IS THE DRIED STAMENS OF A TYPE OF CROCUS FLOWER. IT IS PRICEY, BUT A LITTLE GOES A LONG WAY. IT ADDS ITS EARTHY, DISTINCTIVE FLAVOR AND GORGEOUS YELLOW HUE TO THIS CRISP-SKINNED ROAST CHICKEN.

- 1 4- to 5-pound whole chicken
- 3 tablespoons olive oil
- 6 cloves garlic, crushed and peeled
- 1½ tablespoons finely shredded lemon peel
- 1 tablespoon fresh thyme
- 1½ teaspoons cracked black pepper
- ½ teaspoon saffron threads
- 2 bay leaves
- 1 lemon, quartered

1. Remove neck and giblets from chicken; discard or save for another use. Rinse chicken body cavity; pat dry with paper towels. Snip any excess skin or fat from chicken.

2. In a food processor combine olive oil, garlic, lemon peel, thyme, pepper, and saffron. Process to form a smooth paste.

3. Using fingers, rub paste over the outside surface of the chicken and the inside cavity. Transfer chicken to a large bowl; cover and refrigerate for at least 8 hours or overnight.

4. Preheat oven to 425°F. Place lemon quarters and bay leaves in chicken cavity. Tie legs together with 100%-cotton kitchen string. Tuck wings under chicken. Insert an oven-going meat thermometer into the inside thigh muscle without touching bone. Place chicken on a rack in a large roasting pan.

5. Roast for 15 minutes. Reduce oven temperature to 375°F. Roast about 1 hour more or until juices run clear and thermometer registers 175°F. Tent chicken with foil. Let stand for 10 minutes before carving.

SPATCHCOCKED CHICKEN WITH JICAMA SLAW

PREP: 40 minutes GRILL: 1 hour 5 minutes STAND: 10 minutes MAKES: 4 servings

"SPATCHCOCK" IS AN OLD COOKING TERM THAT'S RECENTLY COME BACK INTO USE TO DESCRIBE THE PROCESS OF SPLITTING A SMALL BIRD—SUCH AS A CHICKEN OR CORNISH HEN—DOWN THE BACK AND THEN OPENING IT AND FLATTENING IT LIKE A BOOK TO HELP IT COOK QUICKLY AND MORE EVENLY. IT'S SIMILAR TO BUTTERFLYING BUT REFERS ONLY TO POULTRY.

CHICKEN
- 1 poblano chile
- 1 tablespoon finely chopped shallot
- 3 cloves garlic, minced
- 1 teaspoon finely shredded lemon peel
- 1 teaspoon finely shredded lime peel
- 1 teaspoon Smoky Seasoning (see recipe)
- ½ teaspoon dried oregano, crushed
- ½ teaspoon ground cumin
- 1 tablespoon olive oil
- 1 3- to 3½-pound whole chicken

SLAW
- ½ of a medium jicama, peeled and cut into julienne strips (about 3 cups)
- ½ cup thinly sliced scallions (4)
- 1 Granny Smith apple, peeled, cored, and cut into julienne strips
- ⅓ cup snipped fresh cilantro
- 3 tablespoons fresh orange juice
- 3 tablespoons olive oil
- 1 teaspoon Lemon-Herb Seasoning (see recipe)

1. For a charcoal grill, arrange medium hot coals on one side of the grill. Place a drip pan under the empty side of the grill. Place poblano on the grill rack directly over medium coals. Cover and grill for 15 minutes or until the poblano is charred on all sides, turning occasionally. Immediately wrap poblano in foil; let stand for 10 minutes. Open foil and cut poblano in half lengthwise; remove stems and seeds (see tip). Using a sharp knife, gently peel off skin and discard. Finely chop the poblano. (For a gas grill, preheat grill; reduce heat to medium. Adjust for indirect cooking. Grill as above over burner that is turned on.)

2. For the rub, in a small bowl combine poblano, shallot, garlic, lemon peel, lime peel, Smoky Seasoning, oregano, and cumin. Stir in oil; mix well to make a paste.

3. To spatchcock the chicken, remove the neck and giblets from chicken (save for another use). Place the chicken, breast side down, on a cutting board. Use kitchen shears to make a lengthwise cut down one side of the backbone, starting from the neck end. Repeat the lengthwise cut to opposite side of the backbone. Remove and discard the backbone. Turn chicken skin side up. Press down between the breasts to break the breast bone so the chicken lies flat.

4. Starting at the neck on one side of the breast, slip your fingers between skin and meat, loosening skin as you work toward the thigh. Free the skin around the thigh. Repeat on the other side. Use your fingers to spread rub over the meat under the skin of the chicken.

5. Place chicken, breast side down, on grill rack over drip pan. Weight with two foil-wrapped bricks or a large cast-iron skillet. Cover and grill for 30 minutes. Turn chicken, bone side down, on rack, weighting again with bricks or skillet. Grill, covered, about 30 minutes more or until chicken is no longer pink (175°F in thigh muscle). Remove chicken from grill; let stand for 10 minutes. (For a gas grill, place chicken on grill rack away from heat. Grill as above.)

6. Meanwhile, for the slaw, in a large bowl combine jicama, scallions, apple, and cilantro. In a small bowl whisk together orange juice, oil, and Lemon-Herb Seasoning. Pour over the jicama mixture and toss to coat. Serve chicken with the slaw.

ROASTED CHICKEN HINDQUARTERS WITH VODKA, CARROT, AND TOMATO SAUCE

PREP: 15 minutes COOK: 15 minutes ROAST: 30 minutes MAKES: 4 servings

VODKA CAN BE MADE FROM SEVERAL DIFFERENT FOODSTUFFS, INCLUDING POTATOES, CORN, RYE, WHEAT, AND BARLEY—EVEN GRAPES. ALTHOUGH THERE ISN'T MUCH VODKA IN THIS SAUCE WHEN YOU DIVIDE IT AMONG FOUR SERVINGS, LOOK FOR VOKDA MADE FROM EITHER POTATOES OR GRAPES TO BE PALEO COMPLIANT.

3 tablespoons olive oil

4 bone-in chicken hindquarters or meaty chicken pieces, skinned

1 28-ounce can no-salt-added plum tomatoes, drained

½ cup finely chopped onion

½ cup finely chopped carrot

3 cloves garlic, minced

1 teaspoon Mediterranean Seasoning (see recipe)

⅛ teaspoon cayenne pepper

1 sprig fresh rosemary

2 tablespoons vodka

1 tablespoon snipped fresh basil (optional)

1. Preheat oven to 375°F. In an extra-large skillet heat 2 tablespoons of the oil over medium-high heat. Add chicken; cook about 12 minutes or until browned, turning to brown evenly. Place skillet in the preheated oven. Roast, uncovered, for 20 minutes.

2. Meanwhile, for sauce, use kitchen scissors to cut up the tomatoes. In a medium saucepan heat the remaining 1

tablespoon oil over medium heat. Add onion, carrot, and garlic; cook for 3 minutes or until tender, stirring frequently. Stir in snipped tomatoes, Mediterranean Seasoning, cayenne pepper, and rosemary sprig. Bring to boiling over medium-high heat; reduce heat. Simmer, uncovered, for 10 minutes, stirring occasionally. Stir in vodka; cook 1 minute more; remove and discard rosemary sprig.

3. Ladle sauce over chicken in skillet. Return skillet to oven. Roast, covered, about 10 minutes more or until chicken is tender and no longer pink (175°F). If desired, sprinkle with basil.

POULET RÔTI AND RUTABAGA FRITES

PREP: 40 minutes BAKE: 40 minutes MAKES: 4 servings

THE CRISP RUTABAGA FRITES ARE DELICIOUS SERVED WITH THE ROASTED CHICKEN AND ITS ATTENDANT COOKING JUICES—BUT THEY ARE EQUALLY TASTY MADE ON THEIR OWN AND SERVED WITH PALEO KETCHUP (SEE RECIPE) OR SERVED BELGIAN-STYLE WITH PALEO AÏOLI (GARLIC MAYO, SEE RECIPE).

- 6 tablespoons olive oil
- 1 tablespoon Mediterranean Seasoning (see recipe)
- 4 bone-in chicken thighs, skinned (about 1 ¼ pounds total)
- 4 chicken drumsticks, skinned (about 1 pound total)
- 1 cup dry white wine
- 1 cup Chicken Bone Broth (see recipe) or no-salt-added chicken broth
- 1 small onion, quartered
- Olive oil
- 1½ to 2 pounds rutabagas
- 2 tablespoons snipped fresh chives
- Black pepper

1. Preheat oven to 400°F. In a small bowl combine 1 tablespoon of the olive oil and the Mediterranean Seasoning; rub onto chicken pieces. In an extra-large oven-going skillet heat 2 tablespoons of the oil. Add chicken pieces, meaty sides down. Cook, uncovered, about 5 minutes or until browned. Remove skillet from heat. Turn chicken pieces, browned sides up. Add wine, Chicken Bone Broth, and onion.

2. Place skillet in oven on middle rack. Bake, uncovered, for 10 minutes.

3. Meanwhile, for frites, lightly brush a large baking sheet with olive oil; set aside. Peel rutabagas. Using a sharp knife, cut rutabagas into ½-inch slices. Cut slices lengthwise into ½-inch strips. In a large bowl toss rutabaga strips with the remaining 3 tablespoons oil. Spread rutabaga strips in a single layer on prepared baking sheet; place in oven on top rack. Bake for 15 minutes; turn frites over. Bake chicken for 10 minutes more or until no longer pink (175°F). Remove chicken from oven. Bake frites 5 to 10 minutes or until browned and tender.

4. Remove chicken and onion from skillet, reserving juices. Cover chicken and onion to keep warm. Bring juices to boiling over medium heat; reduce heat. Simmer, uncovered, about 5 minutes more or until juices are slightly reduced.

5. To serve, toss frites with chives and season with pepper. Serve chicken with cooking juices and frites.

TRIPLE-MUSHROOM COQ AU VIN WITH CHIVE MASHED RUTABAGAS

PREP: 15 minutes COOK: 1 hour 15 minutes MAKES: 4 to 6 servings

IF THERE IS ANY GRIT IN THE BOWL AFTER SOAKING THE DRIED MUSHROOMS—AND IT IS LIKELY THAT THERE WILL BE—STRAIN THE LIQUID THROUGH A DOUBLE THICKNESS OF CHEESECLOTH SET IN A FINE-MESH STRAINER.

- 1 ounce dried porcini or morel mushrooms
- 1 cup boiling water
- 2 to 2½ pounds chicken thighs and drumsticks, skinned
- Black pepper
- 2 tablespoons olive oil
- 2 medium leeks, halved lengthwise, rinsed, and thinly sliced
- 2 portobello mushrooms, sliced
- 8 ounces fresh oyster mushrooms, stemmed and sliced, or sliced fresh button mushrooms
- ¼ cup no-salt-added tomato paste
- 1 teaspoon dried marjoram, crushed
- ½ teaspoon dried thyme, crushed
- ½ cup dry red wine
- 6 cups Chicken Bone Broth (see recipe) or no-salt-added chicken broth
- 2 bay leaves
- 2 to 2½ pounds rutabagas, peeled and chopped
- 2 tablespoons snipped fresh chives
- ½ teaspoon black pepper
- Snipped fresh thyme (optional)

1. In a small bowl combine the porcini mushrooms and the boiling water; let stand for 15 minutes. Remove mushrooms, reserving the soaking liquid. Chop the mushrooms. Set the mushrooms and soaking liquid aside.

2. Sprinkle chicken with pepper. In an extra-large skillet with a tight-fitting lid heat 1 tablespoon of the olive oil over medium-high heat. Cook chicken pieces, in two batches, in hot oil about 15 minutes until lightly browned, turning once. Remove chicken from the skillet. Stir in leeks, portobello mushrooms, and oyster mushrooms. Cook for 4 to 5 minutes or just until mushrooms start to brown, stirring occasionally. Stir in tomato paste, marjoram, and thyme; cook and stir for 1 minute. Stir in wine; cook and stir for 1 minute. Stir in 3 cups of the Chicken Bone Broth, bay leaves, ½ cup of the reserved mushroom soaking liquid, and rehydrated chopped mushrooms. Return chicken to skillet. Bring to boiling; reduce heat. Simmer, covered, about 45 minutes or until chicken is tender, turning the chicken once halfway through cooking.

3. Meanwhile, in a large saucepan combine rutabagas and the remaining 3 cups broth. If necessary, add water to just cover rutabagas. Bring to boiling; reduce heat. Simmer, uncovered, for 25 to 30 minutes or until rutabagas are tender, stirring occasionally. Drain rutabagas, reserving liquid. Return rutabagas to the saucepan. Add the remaining 1 tablespoon olive oil, the chives, and the ½ teaspoon pepper. Using a potato masher, mash the rutabaga mixture, adding cooking liquid as needed to make desired consistency.

4. Remove bay leaves from chicken mixture; discard. Serve chicken and sauce over mashed rutabagas. If desired, sprinkle with fresh thyme.

PEACH-BRANDY-GLAZED DRUMSTICKS

PREP: 30 minutes GRILL: 40 minutes MAKES: 4 servings

THESE CHICKEN LEGS ARE PERFECT WITH A CRISPY SLAW AND THE SPICY OVEN-BAKED SWEET POTATO FRIES FROM THE RECIPE FOR TUNISIAN SPICE-RUBBED PORK SHOULDER (SEE RECIPE). THEY'RE SHOWN HERE WITH CRUNCHY CABBAGE SLAW WITH RADISHES, MANGO, AND MINT (SEE RECIPE).

PEACH-BRANDY GLAZE
- 1 tablespoon olive oil
- ½ cup chopped onion
- 2 fresh medium peaches, halved, pitted, and chopped
- 2 tablespoons brandy
- 1 cup BBQ Sauce (see recipe)

8 chicken drumsticks (2 to 2½ pounds total), skinned if desired

1. For glaze, in a medium saucepan heat olive oil over medium heat. Add onion; cook about 5 minutes or until tender, stirring occasionally. Add peaches. Cover and cook for 4 to 6 minutes or until peaches are tender, stirring occasionally. Add brandy; cook, uncovered, for 2 minutes, stirring occasionally. Cool slightly. Transfer peach mixture to a blender or food processor. Cover and blend or process until smooth. Add BBQ Sauce. Cover and blend or process until smooth. Return sauce to the saucepan. Cook over medium-low heat just until heated through. Transfer ¾ cup of the sauce to a small bowl for brushing on the chicken. Keep remaining sauce warm for serving with grilled chicken.

2. For a charcoal grill, arrange medium-hot coals around a drip pan. Test for medium heat above drip pan. Place chicken drumsticks on grill rack over drip pan. Cover and grill for 40 to 50 minutes or until chicken is no longer pink (175°F), turning once halfway through grilling and brushing with ¾ cup of the Peach-Brandy Glaze for the last 5 to 10 minutes of grilling. (For a gas grill, preheat grill. Reduce heat to medium. Adjust heat for indirect cooking. Add chicken drumsticks to grill rack that is not over the heat. Cover and grill as directed.)

CHILE-MARINATED CHICKEN WITH MANGO-MELON SALAD

PREP: 40 minutes CHILL/MARINATE: 2 to 4 hours GRILL: 50 minutes MAKES: 6 to 8 servings

AN ANCHO CHILE IS A DRIED POBLANO—A GLOSSY, DEEP-GREEN CHILE WITH AN INTENSELY FRESH FLAVOR. ANCHO CHILES HAVE A SLIGHTLY FRUITY FLAVOR WITH A HINT OF PLUM OR RAISIN AND JUST A TOUCH OF BITTERNESS. NEW MEXICO CHILES CAN BE MODERATELY HOT. THEY'RE THE DEEP-RED CHILES YOU SEE BUNCHED AND HANGING IN RISTRAS—COLORFUL ARRANGEMENTS OF DRYING CHILES—IN PARTS OF THE SOUTHWEST.

CHICKEN
- 2 dried New Mexico chiles
- 2 dried ancho chiles
- 1 cup boiling water
- 3 tablespoons olive oil
- 1 large sweet onion, peeled and cut into thick slices
- 4 roma tomatoes, cored
- 1 tablespoon minced garlic (6 cloves)
- 2 teaspoons ground cumin
- 1 teaspoon dried oregano, crushed
- 16 chicken drumsticks

SALAD
- 2 cups cubed cantaloupe
- 2 cups cubed honeydew
- 2 cups cubed mango
- ¼ cup fresh lime juice
- 1 teaspoon chili powder

½ teaspoon ground cumin

¼ cup snipped fresh cilantro

1. For chicken, remove stems and seeds from dried New Mexico and ancho chiles. Heat a large skillet over medium heat. Toast chiles in the skillet for 1 to 2 minutes or until fragrant and lightly toasted. Place toasted chiles in a small bowl; add the boiling water to the bowl. Let stand at least 10 minutes or until ready to use.

2. Preheat the broiler. Line a baking sheet with foil; brush 1 tablespoon of the olive oil over foil. Place onion slices and tomatoes on pan. Broil about 4 inches from heat for 6 to 8 minutes or until softened and charred. Drain chiles, reserving the water.

3. For marinade, in a blender or food processor combine chiles, onion, tomatoes, garlic, cumin, and oregano. Cover and blend or process until smooth, adding reserved water as needed to puree and reach desired consistency.

4. Place chicken in a large resealable plastic bag set in a shallow dish. Pour marinade over chicken in bag, turning bag to coat evenly. Marinate in refrigerator for 2 to 4 hours, turning bag occasionally.

5. For salad, in an extra-large bowl combine cantaloupe, honeydew, mango, lime juice, the remaining 2 tablespoons olive oil, chili powder, cumin, and cilantro. Toss to coat. Cover and chill for 1 to 4 hours.

6. For a charcoal grill, arrange medium-hot coals around a drip pan. Test for medium heat above the pan. Drain chicken, reserving the marinade. Place chicken on the grill rack over the drip pan. Brush chicken generously with some of

the reserved marinade (discard any extra marinade). Cover and grill for 50 minutes or until chicken is no longer pink (175°F), turning once halfway through grilling. (For a gas grill, preheat grill. Reduce heat to medium. Adjust for indirect cooking. Continue as directed, placing chicken on the burner that is turned off.) Serve chicken drumsticks with salad.

TANDOORI-STYLE CHICKEN LEGS WITH CUCUMBER RAITA

PREP: 20 minutes MARINATE: 2 to 24 hours BROIL: 25 minutes MAKES: 4 servings

THE RAITA IS MADE WITH CASHEW CREAM, LEMON JUICE, MINT, CILANTRO, AND CUCUMBER. IT PROVIDES A COOLING COUNTERPOINT TO THE HOT AND SPICY CHICKEN.

CHICKEN

- 1 onion, cut into thin wedges
- 1 2-inch piece fresh ginger, peeled and quartered
- 4 cloves garlic
- 3 tablespoons olive oil
- 2 tablespoons fresh lemon juice
- 1 teaspoon ground cumin
- 1 teaspoon ground turmeric
- ½ teaspoon ground allspice
- ½ teaspoon ground cinnamon
- ½ teaspoon black pepper
- ¼ teaspoon cayenne pepper
- 8 chicken drumsticks

CUCUMBER RAITA

- 1 cup Cashew Cream (see [recipe](#))
- 1 tablespoon fresh lemon juice
- 1 tablespoon snipped fresh mint
- 1 tablespoon snipped fresh cilantro
- ½ teaspoon ground cumin
- ⅛ teaspoon black pepper
- 1 medium cucumber, peeled, seeded, and diced (1 cup)
- Lemon wedges

1. In a blender or food processor combine onion, ginger, garlic, olive oil, lemon juice, cumin, turmeric, allspice, cinnamon, black pepper, and cayenne pepper. Cover and blend or process until smooth.

2. Using the tip of a paring knife, pierce each drumstick four or five times. Place drumsticks in a large resealable plastic bag set in a large bowl. Add onion mixture; turn to coat. Marinate in the refrigerator for 2 to 24 hours, turning bag occasionally.

3. Preheat broiler. Remove chicken from marinade. Using paper towels, wipe excess marinade from drumsticks. Arrange drumsticks on the rack of an unheated broiler pan or rimmed baking sheet lined with foil. Broil 6 to 8 inches from heat source for 15 minutes. Turn drumsticks over; broil about 10 minutes or until chicken is no longer pink (175°F).

4. For the raita, in a medium bowl combine Cashew Cream, lemon juice, mint, cilantro, cumin, and black pepper. Gently stir in cucumber.

5. Serve chicken with raita and lemon wedges.

CURRIED CHICKEN STEW WITH ROOT VEGETABLES, ASPARAGUS, AND GREEN APPLE-MINT RELISH

PREP: 30 minutes COOK: 35 minutes STAND: 5 minutes MAKES: 4 servings

2 tablespoons refined coconut oil or olive oil

2 pounds bone-in chicken breasts, skinned if desired

1 cup chopped onion

2 tablespoons grated fresh ginger

2 tablespoons minced garlic

2 tablespoons salt-free curry powder

2 tablespoons minced, seeded jalapeño (see tip)

4 cups Chicken Bone Broth (see recipe) or no-salt-added chicken broth

2 medium sweet potatoes (about 1 pound), peeled and chopped

2 medium turnips (about 6 ounces), peeled and chopped

1 cup seeded, diced tomato

8 ounces asparagus, trimmed and cut into 1-inch lengths

1 13.5-ounce can natural coconut milk (such as Nature's Way)

½ cup snipped fresh cilantro

Apple-Mint Relish (see recipe, below)

Lime wedges

1. In a 6-quart Dutch oven heat oil over medium-high heat. Brown chicken in batches in hot oil, turning to brown evenly, about 10 minutes. Transfer chicken to a plate; set aside.

2. Turn heat to medium. Add onion, ginger, garlic, curry powder, and jalapeño to the pot. Cook and stir 5 minutes or until onion is softened. Stir in Chicken Bone Broth, sweet potatoes, turnips, and tomato. Return the chicken pieces to the pot, arranging to submerge chicken in as much liquid as possible. Reduce heat to medium-low.

Cover and simmer 30 minutes or until chicken is no longer pink and vegetables are tender. Stir in asparagus, coconut milk, and cilantro. Remove from heat. Let stand for 5 minutes. Cut chicken from bones, if necessary, to divide evenly among serving bowls. Serve with Apple-Mint Relish and lime wedges.

Apple-Mint Relish: In a food processor chop ½ cup unsweetened coconut flakes until powdery. Add 1 cup fresh cilantro leaves and steams; 1 cup fresh mint leaves; 1 Granny Smith apple, cored and chopped; 2 teaspoons minced, seeded jalapeño (see tip); and 1 tablespoon fresh lime juice. Pulse until finely minced.

GRILLED CHICKEN PAILLARD SALAD WITH RASPBERRIES, BEETS, AND ROASTED ALMONDS

PREP: 30 minutes ROAST: 45 minutes MARINATE: 15 minutes GRILL: 8 minutes MAKES: 4 servings

- ½ cup whole almonds
- 1½ teaspoons olive oil
- 1 medium red beet
- 1 medium golden beet
- 2 6- to 8-ounce boneless, skinless chicken breast halves
- 2 cups fresh or frozen raspberries, thawed
- 3 tablespoons white or red wine vinegar
- 2 tablespoons snipped fresh tarragon
- 1 tablespoon minced shallot
- 1 teaspoon Dijon-Style Mustard (see recipe)
- ¼ cup olive oil
- Black pepper
- 8 cups spring mix lettuces

1. For the almonds, preheat the oven to 400°F. Spread almonds on a small baking sheet and toss with ½ teaspoon olive oil. Bake about 5 minutes or until fragrant and golden. Let cool. (Almonds may be toasted 2 days ahead and stored in an airtight container.)

2. For the beets, place each beet on a small piece of foil and drizzle with each with ½ teaspoon olive oil. Loosely wrap the foil around the beets and place on a baking sheet or in a baking dish. Roast the beets in the 400°F oven for 40 to 50 minutes or until tender when pierced with a knife. Remove from oven and let stand until cool enough to handle. Using a paring knife, remove the skin. Cut beets

into wedges and set aside. (Avoid mixing the beets together to prevent the red beets from staining the golden beets. Beets may be roasted 1 day ahead and chilled. Bring to room temperature before serving.)

3. For the chicken, cut each chicken breast in half horizontally. Place each piece of chicken between two pieces of plastic wrap. Using a meat mallet, gently pound to about ¾ inch thick. Place chicken in a shallow dish and set aside.

4. For vinaigrette, in a large bowl lightly crush ¾ cup of the raspberries with a whisk (reserve remaining raspberries for the salad). Add the vinegar, tarragon, shallot, and Dijon-Style Mustard; whisk to blend. Add the ¼ cup olive oil in a thin stream, whisking to mix well. Pour ½ cup vinaigrette over the chicken; turn chicken to coat (reserve remaining vinaigrette for the salad). Marinate chicken at room temperature for 15 minutes. Remove chicken from the marinade and sprinkle with pepper; discard marinade remaining in dish.

5. For a charcoal or gas grill, place chicken on a grill rack directly over medium heat. Cover and grill for 8 to 10 minutes or until chicken is no longer pink, turning once halfway through grilling. (Chicken can also be cooked in a stovetop grill pan.)

6. In a large bowl combine lettuce, beets, and the remaining 1¼ cups raspberries. Pour reserved vinaigrette over salad; gently toss to coat. Divide salad among four serving plates; top each with a grilled chicken breast piece. Coarsely chop the roasted almonds and sprinkle over all. Serve immediately.

BROCCOLI RABE-STUFFED CHICKEN BREASTS WITH FRESH TOMATO SAUCE AND CAESAR SALAD

PREP: 40 minutes COOK: 25 minutes MAKES: 6 servings

3 tablespoons olive oil

2 teaspoons minced garlic

¼ teaspoon crushed red pepper

1 pound broccoli raab, trimmed and chopped

½ cup unsulfured golden raisins

½ cup water

4 5- to 6-ounce skinless, boneless chicken breast halves

1 cup chopped onion

3 cups chopped tomatoes

¼ cup snipped fresh basil

2 teaspoons red wine vinegar

3 tablespoons fresh lemon juice

2 tablespoons Paleo Mayo (see recipe)

2 teaspoons Dijon-Style Mustard (see recipe)

1 teaspoon minced garlic

½ teaspoon black pepper

¼ cup olive oil

10 cups chopped romaine lettuce

1. In a large skillet heat 1 tablespoon of the olive oil over medium-high heat. Add the garlic and crushed red pepper; cook and stir for 30 seconds or until fragrant. Add the chopped broccoli rabe, raisins, and the ½ cup water. Cover and cook about 8 minutes or until broccoli raab is wilted and tender. Remove lid from pan; let any excess water evaporate. Set aside.

2. For roulades, halve each chicken breast lengthwise; place each piece between two pieces of plastic wrap. Using the flat side of a meat mallet, pound chicken lightly to about ¼ inch thick. For each roulade, place about ¼ cup of the broccoli raab mixture on one of the short ends; roll up, folding in the sides to completely enclose filling. (Roulades may be made up to 1 day ahead and chilled until ready to cook.)

3. In a large skillet heat 1 tablespoon of the olive oil over medium-high heat. Add the roulades, seam sides down. Cook about 8 minutes or until browned on all sides, turning two or three times during cooking. Transfer roulades to a platter.

4. For sauce, in the skillet heat 1 tablespoon of the remaining olive oil over medium heat. Add the onion; cook about 5 minutes or until translucent. Stir in the tomatoes and basil. Place roulades on top of the sauce in skillet. Bring to boiling over medium-high heat; reduce heat. Cover and simmer about 5 minutes or until tomatoes start to break down but still retain their shape and roulades are heated through.

5. For dressing, in a small bowl whisk together the lemon juice, Paleo Mayo, Dijon-Style Mustard, garlic, and black pepper. Drizzle in the ¼ cup olive oil, whisking until emulsified. In a large bowl toss dressing with the chopped romaine. To serve, divide romaine among six serving plates. Slice roulades and arrange on romaine; drizzle with tomato sauce.

GRILLED CHICKEN SHAWARMA WRAPS WITH SPICED VEGETABLES AND PINE NUT DRESSING

PREP: 20 minutes MARINATE: 30 minutes GRILL: 10 minutes MAKES: 8 wraps (4 servings)

1½ pounds skinless, boneless chicken breast halves, cut into 2-inch pieces
5 tablespoons olive oil
2 tablespoons fresh lemon juice
1¾ teaspoons ground cumin
1 teaspoon minced garlic
1 teaspoon paprika
½ teaspoon curry powder
½ teaspoon ground cinnamon
¼ teaspoon cayenne pepper
1 medium zucchini, halved
1 small eggplant cut into ½-inch slices
1 large yellow sweet pepper, halved and seeded
1 medium red onion, quartered
8 cherry tomatoes
8 large butter lettuce leaves
Toasted Pine Nut Dressing (see recipe)
Lemon wedges

1. For marinade, in a small bowl combine 3 tablespoons of the olive oil, lemon juice, 1 teaspoon of the cumin, garlic, ½ teaspoon of the paprika, curry powder, ¼ teaspoon of the cinnamon, and cayenne pepper. Place chicken pieces in a large resealable plastic bag set in a shallow dish. Pour marinade over the chicken. Seal bag; turn bag to coat. Marinate in the refrigerator for 30 minutes, turning bag occasionally.

2. Remove chicken from marinade; discard marinade. Thread chicken on four long skewers.

3. Place zucchini, eggplant, sweet pepper, and onion on a baking sheet. Drizzle with 2 tablespoons of the olive oil. Sprinkle with the remaining ¾ teaspoon cumin, remaining ½ teaspoon paprika, and the remaining ¼ teaspoon cinnamon; lightly rub over vegetables. Thread tomatoes on two skewers.

3. For a charcoal or gas grill, place chicken and tomato kabobs and vegetables on a grill rack over medium heat. Cover and grill until chicken is no longer pink and vegetables are lightly charred and crisp-tender, turning once. Allow 10 to 12 minutes for chicken, 8 to 10 minutes for vegetables, and 4 minutes for tomatoes.

4. Remove chicken from skewers. Chop chicken and cut zucchini, eggplant, and sweet pepper into bite-size pieces. Remove the tomatoes from skewers (do not chop). Arrange chicken and vegetables on a platter. To serve, spoon some of the chicken and vegetables into a lettuce leaf; drizzle with Toasted Pine Nut Dressing. Serve with lemon wedges.

OVEN-BRAISED CHICKEN BREASTS WITH MUSHROOMS, GARLIC-MASHED CAULIFLOWER, AND ROASTED ASPARAGUS

START TO FINISH: 50 minutes MAKES: 4 servings

4 10- to 12-ounce bone-in chicken breast halves, skinned

3 cups small white button mushrooms

1 cup thinly sliced leeks or yellow onion

2 cups Chicken Bone Broth (see recipe) or no-salt-added chicken broth

1 cup dry white wine

1 large bunch fresh thyme

Black pepper

White wine vinegar (optional)

1 head cauliflower, separated into florets

12 cloves garlic, peeled

2 tablespoons olive oil

White or cayenne pepper

1 pound asparagus, trimmed

2 teaspoons olive oil

1. Preheat oven to 400°F. Arrange chicken breasts in a 3-quart rectangular baking dish; top with mushrooms and leeks. Pour Chicken Bone Broth and wine over the chicken and vegetables. Scatter thyme over all and sprinkle with black pepper. Cover dish with foil.

2. Bake for 35 to 40 minutes or until an instant-read thermometer inserted in chicken registers 170°F. Remove and discard thyme sprigs. If desired, season braising liquid with a splash of vinegar before serving.

2. Meanwhile, in a large saucepan cook cauliflower and garlic in enough boiling water to cover about 10 minutes or until very tender. Drain cauliflower and garlic, reserving 2 tablespoons of the cooking liquid. In a food processor or a large mixing bowl place cauliflower and reserved cooking liquid. Process until smooth* or mash with a potato masher; stir in 2 tablespoons olive oil and season to taste with white pepper. Keep warm until ready to serve.

3. Arrange asparagus in a single layer on a baking sheet. Drizzle with 2 teaspoons olive oil and toss to coat. Sprinkle with black pepper. Roast in a 400°F oven about 8 minutes or until crisp-tender, stirring once.

4. Divide mashed cauliflower among six serving plates. Top with chicken, mushrooms, and leeks. Drizzle with some of the braising liquid; serve with roasted asparagus.

*Note: If using a food processor, be careful not to overprocess or cauliflower will get too thin.

THAI-STYLE CHICKEN SOUP

PREP: 30 minutes FREEZE: 20 minutes COOK: 50 minutes MAKES: 4 to 6 servings

TAMARIND IS A MUSKY, SOUR FRUIT USED IN INDIAN, THAI, AND MEXICAN COOKING. MANY COMMERCIALLY PREPARED TAMARIND PASTES CONTAIN SUGAR—BE SURE YOU PURCHASE ONE THAT DOES NOT. KAFFIR LIME LEAVES CAN BE FOUND FRESH, FROZEN, AND DRIED AT MOST ASIAN MARKETS. IF YOU CAN'T FIND THEM, SUBSTITUTE 1½ TEASPOONS FINELY SHREDDED LIME PEEL FOR THE LEAVES IN THIS RECIPE.

- 2 stalks lemongrass, trimmed
- 2 tablespoons unrefined coconut oil
- ½ cup thinly sliced scallions
- 3 large cloves garlic, thinly sliced
- 8 cups Chicken Bone Broth (see recipe) or no-salt-added chicken broth
- ¼ cup no-sugar-added tamarind paste (such as Tamicon brand)
- 2 tablespoons nori flakes
- 3 fresh Thai chiles, thinly sliced with seeds intact (see tip)
- 3 kaffir lime leaves
- 1 3-inch piece ginger, thinly sliced
- 4 6-ounce skinless, boneless chicken breast halves
- 1 14.5-ounce can no-salt-added fire-roasted diced tomatoes, undrained
- 6 ounces thin asparagus spears, trimmed and thinly sliced diagonally into ½-inch pieces
- ½ cup packed Thai basil leaves (see note)

1. Using the back of a knife with firm pressure, bruise the lemongrass stalks. Finely chop bruised stalks.

2. In a Dutch oven heat coconut oil over medium heat. Add lemongrass and scallions; cook for 8 to 10 minutes,

stirring often. Add garlic; cook and stir for 2 to 3 minutes or until very fragrant.

3. Add Chicken Bone Broth, tamarind paste, nori flakes, chiles, lime leaves, and ginger. Bring to boiling; reduce heat. Cover and simmer for 40 minutes.

4. Meanwhile, freeze chicken for 20 to 30 minutes or until firm. Thinly slice chicken.

5. Strain soup through a fine-mesh sieve into a large saucepan, pressing with the back of a large spoon to extract flavors. Discard solids. Bring soup to boiling. Stir in chicken, undrained tomatoes, asparagus, and basil. Reduce heat; simmer, uncovered, for 2 to 3 minutes or until chicken is cooked through. Serve immediately.

LEMON AND SAGE ROASTED CHICKEN WITH ENDIVE

PREP: 15 minutes ROAST: 55 minutes STAND: 5 minutes MAKES: 4 servings

THE LEMON SLICES AND SAGE LEAF PLACED UNDER THE SKIN OF THE CHICKEN FLAVOR THE MEAT AS IT COOKS—AND MAKE AN EYE-CATCHING DESIGN UNDER THE CRISP, OPAQUE SKIN AFTER IT COMES OUT OF THE OVEN.

4 bone-in chicken breast halves (with skin)
1 lemon, very thinly sliced
4 large sage leaves
2 teaspoons olive oil
2 teaspoons Mediterranean Seasoning (see <u>recipe</u>)
½ teaspoon black pepper
2 tablespoons extra virgin olive oil
2 shallots, sliced
2 cloves garlic, minced
4 heads endive, halved lengthwise

1. Preheat oven to 400°F. Using a paring knife, very carefully loosen the skin from each breast half, leaving it attached on one side. Place 2 lemon slices and 1 sage leaf on the meat of each breast. Gently pull skin back into place and press gently to secure it.

2. Arrange chicken in a shallow roasting pan. Brush chicken with 2 teaspoons olive oil; sprinkle with Mediterranean Seasoning and ¼ teaspoon of the pepper. Roast, uncovered, about 55 minutes or until skin is browned and crisp and an instant-read thermometer inserted into

chicken registers 170°F. Let chicken stand for 10 minutes before serving.

3. Meanwhile, in a large skillet heat the 2 tablespoons olive oil over medium heat. Add shallots; cook about 2 minutes or until translucent. Sprinkle endive with the remaining ¼ teaspoon pepper. Add garlic to skillet. Place endive in skillet, cut sides down. Cook about 5 minutes or until browned. Carefully turn endive over; cook for 2 to 3 minutes more or until tender. Serve with chicken.

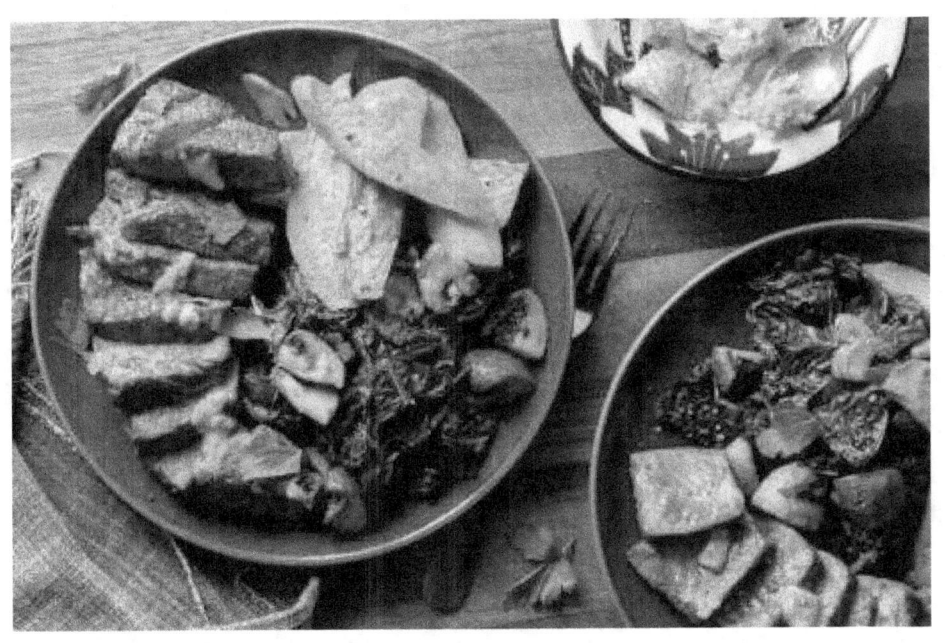

CHICKEN WITH SCALLIONS, WATERCRESS, AND RADISHES

PREP: 20 minutes COOK: 8 minutes BAKE: 30 minutes MAKES: 4 servings

ALTHOUGH IT MIGHT SOUND ODD TO COOK RADISHES, THEY ARE BARELY COOKED HERE—JUST ENOUGH TO MELLOW THEIR PEPPERY BITE AND TENDERIZE THEM A BIT.

- 3 tablespoons olive oil
- 4 10- to 12-ounce bone-in chicken breast halves (with skin)
- 1 tablespoon Lemon-Herb Seasoning (see recipe)
- ¾ cup sliced scallions
- 6 radishes, thinly sliced
- ¼ teaspoon black pepper
- ½ cup dry white vermouth or dry white wine
- ⅓ cup Cashew Cream (see recipe)
- 1 bunch watercress, stems trimmed, roughly chopped
- 1 tablespoon snipped fresh dill

1. Preheat oven to 350°F. In a large skillet heat olive oil over medium-high heat. Pat chicken dry with a paper towel. Cook chicken, skin sides down, for 4 to 5 minutes or until skin is golden and crisp. Turn chicken over; cook about 4 minutes or until browned. Arrange chicken, skin sides up, in a shallow baking dish. Sprinkle chicken with Lemon-Herb Seasoning. Bake about 30 minutes or until an instant-read thermometer inserted into chicken registers 170°F.

2. Meanwhile, pour all but 1 tablespoon drippings from skillet; return skillet to heat. Add scallions and radishes; cook about 3 minutes or just until scallions wilt. Sprinkle with

pepper. Add vermouth, stirring to scrape up browned bits. Bring to boiling; cook until reduced and slightly thickened. Stir in Cashew Cream; bring to boiling. Remove skillet from heat; add watercress and dill, stirring gently just until watercress wilts. Stir in any chicken juices that have accumulated in the baking dish.

3. Divide scallion mixture among four serving plates; top with chicken.

CHICKEN TIKKA MASALA

PREP: 30 minutes MARINATE: 4 to 6 hours COOK: 15 minutes BROIL: 8 minutes MAKES: 4 servings

THIS WAS INSPIRED BY A VERY POPULAR INDIAN DISH THAT MAY NOT HAVE BEEN CREATED IN INDIA AT ALL, BUT RATHER AT AN INDIAN RESTAURANT IN THE UNITED KINGDOM. TRADITIONAL CHICKEN TIKKA MASALA CALLS FOR CHICKEN TO BE MARINATED IN YOGURT AND THEN COOKED IN A SPICY TOMATO SAUCE SPLASHED WITH CREAM. WITHOUT ANY DAIRY BLUNTING THE FLAVOR OF THE SAUCE, THIS VERSION IS ESPECIALLY CLEAN-TASTING. INSTEAD OF RICE, IT'S SERVED OVER CRISP ZUCCHINI NOODLES.

1½ pounds skinless, boneless chicken thighs or chicken breast halves

¾ cup natural coconut milk (such as Nature's Way)

6 cloves garlic, minced

1 tablespoon grated fresh ginger

1 teaspoon ground coriander

1 teaspoon paprika

1 teaspoon ground cumin

¼ teaspoon ground cardamom

4 tablespoons refined coconut oil

1 cup chopped carrots

1 thinly sliced celery

½ cup chopped onion

2 jalapeño or serrano chiles, seeded (if desired) and finely chopped (see tip)

1 14.5-ounce can no-salt-added fire-roasted diced tomatoes, undrained

1 8-ounce can no-salt-added tomato sauce

1 teaspoon no-salt-added garam masala

3 medium zucchini

½ teaspoon black pepper

Fresh cilantro leaves

1. If using chicken thighs, cut each thigh into three pieces. If using chicken breast halves, cut each breast half into 2-inch pieces, cutting any thick portions in half horizontally to make them thinner. Place chicken in a large resealable plastic bag; set aside. For marinade, in a small bowl combine ½ cup of the coconut milk, the garlic, ginger, coriander, paprika, cumin, and cardamom. Pour marinade over chicken in bag. Seal bag and turn to coat chicken. Place bag in a medium bowl; marinate in the refrigerator for 4 to 6 hours, turning bag occasionally.

2. Preheat broiler. In a large skillet heat 2 tablespoons of the coconut oil over medium heat. Add carrots, celery, and onion; cook for 6 to 8 minutes or until vegetables are tender, stirring occasionally. Add jalapeños; cook and stir for 1 minute more. Add undrained tomatoes and tomato sauce. Bring to boiling; reduce heat. Simmer, uncovered, about 5 minutes or until sauce thickens slightly.

3. Drain chicken, discarding marinade. Arrange chicken pieces in a single layer on the unheated rack of a broiler pan. Broil 5 to 6 inches from the heat for 8 to 10 minutes or until chicken is no longer pink, turning once halfway through broiling. Add cooked chicken pieces and the remaining ¼ cup coconut milk to tomato mixture in skillet. Cook for 1 to 2 minutes or until heated through. Remove from the heat; stir in garam masala.

4. Trim ends off zucchini. Using a julienne cutter, cut zucchini into long thin strips. In an extra-large skillet heat the remaining 2 tablespoons coconut oil over medium-high

heat. Add zucchini strips and black pepper. Cook and stir for 2 to 3 minutes or until zucchini is crisp-tender.

5. To serve, divide zucchini among four serving plates. Top with chicken mixture. Garnish with cilantro leaves.

RAS EL HANOUT CHICKEN THIGHS

PREP: 20 minutes COOK: 40 minutes MAKES: 4 servings

RAS EL HANOUT IS A COMPLEX AND EXOTIC MORROCAN SPICE MIXTURE. THE PHRASE MEANS "HEAD OF THE SHOP" IN ARABIC, WHICH IMPLIES THAT IT IS A UNIQUE BLEND OF THE BEST SPICES THE SPICE SELLER HAS TO OFFER. THERE'S NO SET RECIPE FOR RAS EL HANOUT, BUT IT OFTEN CONTAINS SOME BLEND OF GINGER, ANISE, CINNAMON, NUTMEG, PEPPERCORNS, CLOVES, CARDAMOM, DRIED FLOWERS (SUCH AS LAVENDER AND ROSE), NIGELLA, MACE, GALANGAL, AND TURMERIC.

1 tablespoon ground cumin

2 teaspoons ground ginger

1½ teaspoons black pepper

1½ teaspoons ground cinnamon

1 teaspoon ground coriander

1 teaspoon cayenne pepper

1 teaspoon ground allspice

½ teaspoon ground cloves

¼ teaspoon ground nutmeg

1 teaspoon saffron threads (optional)

4 tablespoons unrefined coconut oil

8 bone-in chicken thighs

1 8-ounce package fresh mushrooms, sliced

1 cup chopped onion

1 cup chopped red, yellow, or green sweet pepper (1 large)

4 roma tomatoes, cored, seeded, and chopped

4 cloves garlic, minced

2 13.5-ounce cans natural coconut milk (such as Nature's Way)

3 to 4 tablespoons fresh lime juice

¼ cup finely snipped fresh cilantro

1. For the ras el hanout, in medium mortar or small bowl combine the cumin, ginger, black pepper, cinnamon, coriander, cayenne pepper, allspice, cloves, nutmeg, and, if desired, saffron. Grind with a pestle or stir with a spoon to mix well. Set aside.

2. In an extra-large skillet heat 2 tablespoons of the coconut oil over medium heat. Sprinkle chicken thighs with 1 tablespoon of the ras el hanout. Add chicken to skillet; cook for 5 to 6 minutes or until browned, turning once halfway through cooking. Remove chicken from skillet; keep warm.

3. In the same skillet heat the remaining 2 tablespoons coconut oil over medium heat. Add mushrooms, onion, sweet pepper, tomatoes, and garlic. Cook and stir about 5 minutes or until vegetables are tender. Stir in coconut milk, lime juice, and 1 tablespoon of the ras el hanout. Return chicken to skillet. Bring to boiling; reduce heat. Simmer, covered, about 30 minutes or until chicken is tender (175°F).

4. Serve chicken, vegetables, and sauce in bowls. Garnish with cilantro.

Note: Store leftover Ras el Hanout in a covered container for up to 1 month.

STAR FRUIT ADOBO CHICKEN THIGHS OVER BRAISED SPINACH

PREP: 40 minutes MARINATE: 4 to 8 hours COOK: 45 minutes MAKES: 4 servings

IF NECESSARY, PAT THE CHICKEN DRY WITH A PAPER TOWEL AFTER IT COMES OUT OF THE MARINADE BEFORE BROWNING IT IN THE SKILLET. ANY LIQUID LEFT ON THE MEAT WILL SPATTER IN THE HOT OIL.

- 8 bone-in chicken thighs (1½ to 2 pounds), skinned
- ¾ cup white or cider vinegar
- ¾ cup fresh orange juice
- ½ cup water
- ¼ cup chopped onion
- ¼ cup snipped fresh cilantro
- 4 cloves garlic, minced
- ½ teaspoon black pepper
- 1 tablespoon olive oil
- 1 star fruit (carambola), sliced
- 1 cup Chicken Bone Broth (see recipe) or no-salt-added chicken broth
- 2 9-ounce packages fresh spinach leaves
- Fresh cilantro leaves (optional)

1. Place chicken in a stainless-steel or enamel Dutch oven; set aside. In a medium bowl combine vinegar, orange juice, the water, onion, ¼ cup snipped cilantro, garlic, and pepper; pour over chicken. Cover and marinate in the refrigerator for 4 to 8 hours.

2. Bring chicken mixture in Dutch oven to boiling over medium-high heat; reduce heat. Cover and simmer for 35 to 40 minutes or until chicken is no longer pink (175°F).

3. In an extra-large skillet heat oil over medium-high heat. With tongs, remove chicken from Dutch oven, shaking gently so cooking liquid drips off; reserve cooking liquid. Brown the chicken on all sides, turning frequently to brown evenly.

4. Meanwhile, for sauce, strain cooking liquid; return to Dutch oven. Bring to boiling. Boil about 4 minutes to reduce and thicken slightly; add star fruit; boil for 1 minute more. Return chicken to the sauce in Dutch oven. Remove from heat; cover to keep warm.

5. Wipe out the skillet. Pour Chicken Bone Broth into skillet. Bring to boiling over medium-high heat; stir in spinach. Reduce heat; simmer for 1 to 2 minutes or until spinach is just wilted, stirring constantly. Using a slotted spoon, transfer spinach to a serving platter. Top with chicken and sauce. If desired, sprinkle with cilantro leaves.

CHICKEN-POBLANO CABBAGE TACOS WITH CHIPOTLE MAYO

PREP: 25 minutes BAKE: 40 minutes MAKES: 4 servings

SERVE THESE MESSY-BUT-TASTY TACOS WITH A FORK TO RETRIEVE ANY OF THE FILLING THAT HAPPENS TO FALL OUT OF THE CABBAGE LEAF WHILE YOU'RE EATING IT.

- 1 tablespoon olive oil
- 2 poblano chiles, seeded (if desired) and chopped (see tip)
- ½ cup chopped onion
- 3 cloves garlic, minced
- 1 tablespoon salt-free chili powder
- 2 teaspoons ground cumin
- ½ teaspoon black pepper
- 1 8-ounce can no-salt-added tomato sauce
- ¾ cup Chicken Bone Broth (see recipe) or no-salt-added chicken broth
- 1 teaspoon dried Mexican oregano, crushed
- 1 to 1½ pounds skinless, boneless chicken thighs
- 10 to 12 medium to large cabbage leaves
- Chipotle Paleo Mayo (see recipe)

1. Preheat oven to 350°F. In a large ovenproof skillet heat oil over medium-high heat. Add poblano chiles, onion, and garlic; cook and stir for 2 minutes. Stir in chili powder, cumin, and black pepper; cook and stir for 1 minute more (if necessary, reduce heat to prevent spices from burning).

2. Add tomato sauce, Chicken Bone Broth, and oregano to skillet. Bring to boiling. Carefully place chicken thighs in the tomato mixture. Cover skillet with lid. Bake about 40 minutes or until chicken is tender (175°F), turning chicken once halfway.

3. Remove chicken from skillet; cool slightly. Using two forks, shred chicken into bite-size pieces. Stir shredded chicken into tomato mixture in skillet.

4. To serve, spoon chicken mixture into cabbage leaves; top with Chipotle Paleo Mayo.

CHICKEN STEW WITH BABY CARROTS AND BOK CHOY

PREP: 15 minutes COOK: 24 minutes STAND: 2 minutes MAKES: 4 servings

BABY BOK CHOY IS VERY DELICATE AND CAN GET OVERCOOKED IN A FLASH. TO KEEP IT CRISP AND FRESH-TASTING—NOT WILTED AND SOGGY—BE SURE IT STEAMS IN THE COVERED HOT POT (OFF THE HEAT) FOR NO MORE THAN 2 MINUTES BEFORE YOU SERVE THE STEW.

- 2 tablespoons olive oil
- 1 leek, sliced (white and light green parts)
- 4 cups Chicken Bone Broth (see recipe) or no-salt-added chicken broth
- 1 cup dry white wine
- 1 tablespoon Dijon-Style Mustard (see recipe)
- ½ teaspoon black pepper
- 1 sprig fresh thyme
- 1¼ pounds skinless, boneless chicken thighs, cut into 1-inch pieces
- 8 ounces baby carrots with tops, scrubbed, trimmed, and halved lengthwise, or 2 medium carrots, bias-sliced
- 2 teaspoons finely shredded lemon peel (set aside)
- 1 tablespoon fresh lemon juice
- 2 heads baby bok choy
- ½ teaspoon snipped fresh thyme

1. In a large saucepan heat 1 tablespoon of the olive oil over medium heat. Cook leek in hot oil for 3 to 4 minutes or until wilted. Add Chicken Bone Broth, wine, Dijon-Style Mustard, ¼ teaspoon of the pepper, and thyme sprig. Bring to boiling; reduce heat. Cook for 10 to 12 minutes or until liquid is reduced by about one-third. Discard thyme sprig.

2. Meanwhile, in a Dutch oven heat the remaining 1 tablespoon olive oil over medium-high heat. Sprinkle chicken with the remaining ¼ teaspoon pepper. Cook in hot oil about 3 minutes or until browned, stirring occasionally. Drain fat if necessary. Carefully add the reduced broth mixture to pot, scraping up any brown bits; add carrots. Bring to boiling; reduce heat. Simmer, uncovered, for 8 to 10 minutes or just until carrots are tender. Stir in lemon juice. Cut bok choy in half lengthwise. (If bok choy heads are large, cut into quarters.) Place bok choy on top of chicken in pot. Cover and remove from heat; let stand for 2 minutes.

3. Ladle stew into shallow bowls. Sprinkle with lemon peel and snipped thyme.

CASHEW-ORANGE CHICKEN AND SWEET PEPPER STIR-FRY IN LETTUCE WRAPS

START TO FINISH: 45 minutes MAKES: 4 to 6 servings

YOU WILL FIND TWO TYPES OF COCONUT OIL ON THE SHELVES—REFINED AND EXTRA VIRGIN, OR UNREFINED. AS THE NAME IMPLIES, EXTRA VIRGIN COCONUT OIL IS FROM THE FIRST PRESSING OF THE FRESH, RAW COCONUT. IT IS ALWAYS THE BETTER CHOICE WHEN YOU ARE COOKING OVER MEDIUM OR MEDIUM-HIGH HEAT. REFINED COCONUT OIL HAS A HIGHER SMOKE POINT, SO USE IT ONLY WHEN YOU ARE COOKING OVER HIGH HEAT.

- 1 tablespoon refined coconut oil
- 1½ to 2 pounds skinless, boneless chicken thighs, cut into thin bite-size strips
- 3 red, orange, and/or yellow sweet peppers, stemmed, seeded, and thinly sliced into bite-size strips
- 1 red onion, halved lengthwise and thinly sliced
- 1 teaspoon finely shredded orange peel (set aside)
- ½ cup fresh orange juice
- 1 tablespoon minced fresh ginger
- 3 cloves garlic, minced
- 1 cup unsalted raw cashews, toasted and coarsely chopped (see tip)
- ½ cup sliced green scallions (4)
- 8 to 10 butter or iceberg lettuce leaves

1. In a wok or large skillet heat the coconut oil over high heat. Add chicken; cook and stir for 2 minutes. Add peppers and onion; cook and stir for 2 to 3 minutes or until vegetables just start to soften. Remove the chicken and vegetables from the wok; keep warm.

2. Wipe out wok with paper towel. Add the orange juice to the wok. Cook about 3 minutes or until juice boils and reduces slightly. Add ginger and garlic. Cook and stir for 1 minute. Return the chicken and pepper mixture to the wok. Stir in orange peel, cashews, and scallions. Serve stir-fry on lettuce leaves.

VIETNAMESE COCONUT-LEMONGRASS CHICKEN

START TO FINISH: 30 minutes MAKES: 4 servings

THIS QUICK COCONUT CURRY CAN BE ON THE TABLE IN 30 MINUTES FROM THE TIME YOU START CHOPPING, MAKING IT AN IDEAL MEAL FOR A BUSY WEEKNIGHT.

- 1 tablespoon unrefined coconut oil
- 4 stalks lemongrass (pale parts only)
- 1 3.2-ounce package oyster mushrooms, chopped
- 1 large onion, thinly sliced, rings halved
- 1 fresh jalapeño, seeded and finely chopped (see tip)
- 2 tablespoons minced fresh ginger
- 3 cloves garlic minced
- 1½ pounds skinless, boneless chicken thighs, thinly sliced and cut into bite-size pieces
- ½ cup natural coconut milk (such as Nature's Way)
- ½ cup Chicken Bone Broth (see recipe) or no-salt-added chicken broth
- 1 tablespoon salt-free red curry powder
- ½ teaspoon black pepper
- ½ cup snipped fresh basil leaves
- 2 tablespoons fresh lime juice
- Unsweetened shaved coconut (optional)

1. In an extra-large skillet heat coconut oil over medium heat. Add lemongrass; cook and stir for 1 minute. Add mushrooms, onion, jalapeño, ginger, and garlic; cook and stir for 2 minutes or until onion is just tender. Add chicken; cook about 3 minutes or until chicken is cooked through.

2. In a small bowl combine coconut milk, Chicken Bone Broth, curry powder, and black pepper. Add to chicken mixture in skillet; cook for 1 minute or until the liquid has slightly thickened. Remove from heat; stir in fresh basil and lime juice. If desired, sprinkle servings with coconut.

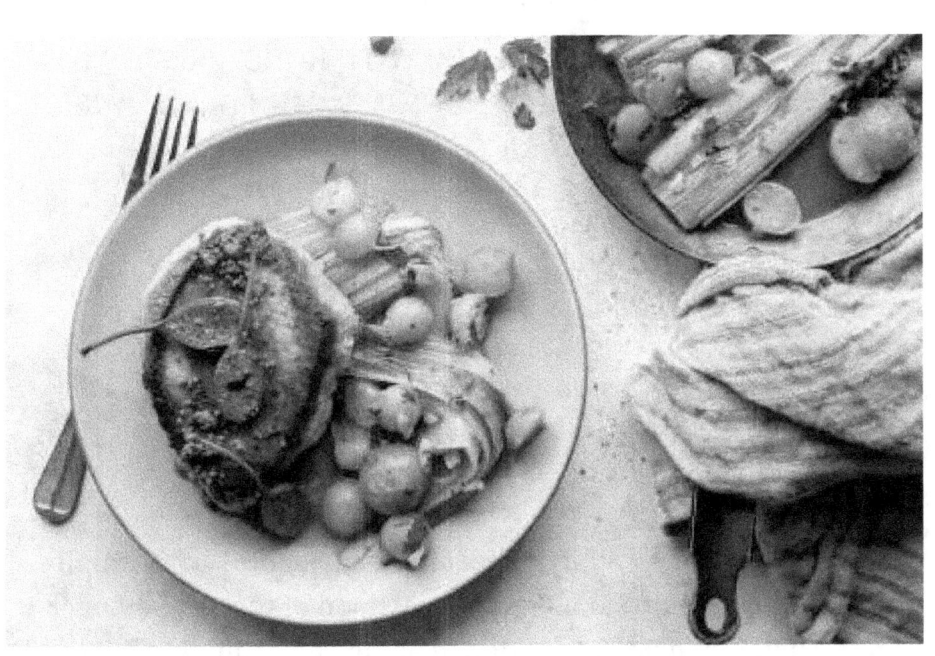

GRILLED CHICKEN AND APPLE ESCAROLE SALAD

PREP: 30 minutes GRILL: 12 minutes MAKES: 4 servings

IF YOU LIKE A SWEETER APPLE, GO WITH HONEYCRISP. IF YOU LIKE A TART APPLE, USE GRANNY SMITH—OR, FOR BALANCE, TRY A MIX OF THE TWO VARIETIES.

- 3 medium Honeycrisp or Granny Smith apples
- 4 teaspoons extra virgin olive oil
- ½ cup finely chopped shallots
- 2 tablespoons snipped fresh parsley
- 1 tablespoon poultry seasoning
- 3 to 4 heads escarole, quartered
- 1 pound ground chicken or turkey breast
- ⅓ cup chopped toasted hazelnuts*
- ⅓ cup Classic French Vinaigrette (see recipe)

1. Halve and core apples. Peel and finely chop 1 of the apples. In a medium skillet heat 1 teaspoon of the olive oil over medium heat. Add chopped apple and shallots; cook until tender. Stir in parsley and poultry seasoning. Set aside to cool.

2. Meanwhile, core the remaining 2 apples and cut into wedges. Brush cut sides of apple wedges and escarole with the remaining olive oil. In a large bowl combine chicken and the cooled apple mixture. Divide into eight portions; shape each portion into a 2-inch-diameter patty.

3. For a charcoal or gas grill, place chicken patties and apple wedges on a grill rack directly over medium heat. Cover and grill for 10 minutes, turning once halfway through

grilling. Add escarole, cut sides down. Cover and grill for 2 to 4 minutes or until escarole is lightly charred, apples are tender, and chicken patties are done (165°F).

4. Coarsely chop escarole. Divide escarole among four serving plates. Top with chicken patties, apple slices, and hazelnuts. Drizzle with Classic French Vinaigrette.

*Tip: To toast hazelnuts, preheat oven to 350°F. Spread nuts in a single layer in a shallow baking pan. Bake for 8 to 10 minutes or until lightly toasted, stirring once to toast evenly. Cool nuts slightly. Place the warm nuts on a clean kitchen towel; rub with the towel to remove the loose skins.

TUSCAN CHICKEN SOUP WITH KALE RIBBONS

PREP: 15 minutes COOK: 20 minutes MAKES: 4 to 6 servings

A SPOONFUL OF PESTO—YOUR CHOICE OF EITHER BASIL OR ARUGULA—ADDS GREAT TASTE TO THIS SAVORY SOUP SEASONED WITH SALT-FREE POULTRY SEASONING. TO KEEP THE KALE RIBBONS BRIGHT GREEN AND AS FULL OF NUTRIENTS AS POSSIBLE, COOK THEM ONLY UNTIL THEY WILT.

- 1 pound ground chicken
- 2 tablespoons no-salt-added poultry seasoning
- 1 teaspoon finely shredded lemon peel
- 1 tablespoon olive oil
- 1 cup chopped onion
- ½ cup chopped carrots
- 1 cup chopped celery
- 4 cloves garlic, sliced
- 4 cups Chicken Bone Broth (see recipe) or no-salt-added chicken broth
- 1 14.5-ounce can no-salt-added fire-roasted tomatoes, undrained
- 1 bunch Lacinato (Tuscan) kale, stems removed, cut into ribbons
- 2 tablespoons fresh lemon juice
- 1 teaspoon snipped fresh thyme
- Basil or Arugula Pesto (see recipes)

1. In a medium bowl combine ground chicken, poultry seasoning, and lemon peel. Mix well.

2. In a Dutch oven heat olive oil over medium heat. Add chicken mixture, onion, carrots, and celery; cook for 5 to 8 minutes or until chicken is no longer pink, stirring with a wooden spoon to break up meat and adding garlic slices the last 1 minute of cooking. Add Chicken Bone Broth and

tomatoes. Bring to boiling; reduce heat. Cover and simmer for 15 minutes. Stir in kale, lemon juice, and thyme. Simmer, uncovered, about 5 minutes or until kale is just wilted.

3. To serve, ladle soup into serving bowls and top with Basil or Arugula Pesto.

CHICKEN LARB

PREP: 15 minutes COOK: 8 minutes COOL: 20 minutes MAKES: 4 servings

THIS VERSION OF THE POPULAR THAI DISH OF HIGHLY SEASONED GROUND CHICKEN AND VEGETABLES SERVED IN LETTUCE LEAVES IS INCREDIBLY LIGHT AND FLAVORFUL—WITHOUT THE ADDITION OF THE SUGAR, SALT, AND FISH SAUCE (WHICH IS VERY HIGH IN SODIUM) THAT ARE TRADITIONALLY PART OF THE INGREDIENTS LIST. WITH GARLIC, THAI CHILES, LEMONGRASS, LIME PEEL, LIME JUICE, MINT, AND CILANTRO, YOU WON'T MISS THEM.

- 1 tablespoon refined coconut oil
- 2 pounds ground chicken (95% lean or ground breast)
- 8 ounces button mushrooms, finely chopped
- 1 cup finely chopped red onion
- 1 to 2 Thai chiles, seeded and finely chopped (see tip)
- 2 tablespoons minced garlic
- 2 tablespoons finely chopped lemongrass*
- ¼ teaspoon ground cloves
- ¼ teaspoon black pepper
- 1 tablespoon finely shredded lime peel
- ½ cup fresh lime juice
- ⅓ cup tightly packed fresh mint leaves, chopped
- ⅓ cup tightly packed fresh cilantro, chopped
- 1 head iceberg lettuce, separated into leaves

1. In an extra-large skillet heat coconut oil over medium-high heat. Add ground chicken, mushrooms, onion, chile(s), garlic, lemongrass, cloves, and black pepper. Cook for 8 to 10 minutes or until chicken is cooked through, stirring with a wooden spoon to break up meat as it cooks. Drain if necessary. Transfer chicken mixture to an extra-large

bowl. Let cool about 20 minutes or until slightly warmer than room temperature, stirring occasionally.

2. Stir lime peel, lime juice, mint, and cilantro into chicken mixture. Serve in lettuce leaves.

*Tip: To prepare the lemongrass, you'll need a sharp knife. Cut the woody stem off of the bottom of the stalk and the tough green blades at the top of the plant. Remove the two tough outer layers. You should have a piece of lemongrass that is about 6 inches long and pale yellow-white. Cut the stalk in half horizontally, then cut each half in half again. Slice each quarter of the stalk very thinly.

CHICKEN BURGERS WITH SZECHWAN CASHEW SAUCE

PREP: 30 minutes COOK: 5 minutes GRILL: 14 minutes MAKES: 4 servings

THE CHILI OIL MADE BY WARMING OLIVE OIL WITH CRUSHED RED PEPPER CAN BE USED IN OTHER WAYS AS WELL. USE IT TO SAUTÉ FRESH VEGETABLES—OR TOSS THEM WITH SOME CHILI OIL BEFORE ROASTING.

- 2 tablespoons olive oil
- ¼ teaspoon crushed red pepper
- 2 cups raw cashew pieces, toasted (see tip)
- ¼ cup olive oil
- ½ cup shredded zucchini
- ¼ cup finely chopped chives
- 2 cloves garlic, minced
- 2 teaspoons finely shredded lemon peel
- 2 teaspoons grated fresh ginger
- 1 pound ground chicken or turkey breast

SZECHWAN CASHEW SAUCE

- 1 tablespoon olive oil
- 2 tablespoons finely chopped scallions
- 1 tablespoon grated fresh ginger
- 1 teaspoon Chinese five-spice powder
- 1 teaspoon fresh lime juice
- 4 green leaf or butter lettuce leaves

1. For the chili oil, in a small saucepan combine the olive oil and the crushed red pepper. Warm over low heat for 5 minutes. Remove from heat; let cool.

2. For cashew butter, place cashews and 1 tablespoon of the olive oil in a blender. Cover and blend until creamy,

stopping to scrape down the sides as needed and adding additional olive oil, 1 tablespoon at a time, until the entire ¼ cup has been used and the butter is very soft; set aside.

3. In a large bowl combine the zucchini, chives, garlic, lemon peel, and the 2 teaspoons ginger. Add ground chicken; mix well. Shape chicken mixture into four ½-inch-thick patties.

4. For a charcoal or gas grill, place patties on the greased rack directly over medium heat. Cover and grill for 14 to 16 minutes or until done (165°F), turning once halfway through grilling.

5. Meanwhile, for the sauce, in a small skillet heat the olive oil over medium heat. Add the scallions and the 1 tablespoon ginger; cook over medium-low heat for 2 minutes or until scallions soften. Add ½ cup of the cashew butter (refrigerate remaining cashew butter for up to 1 week), chili oil, lime juice, and five-spice powder. Cook for 2 more minutes. Remove from heat.

6. Serve patties on the lettuce leaves. Drizzle with sauce.

TURKISH CHICKEN WRAPS

PREP: 25 minutes STAND: 15 minutes COOK: 8 minutes MAKES: 4 to 6 servings

"BAHARAT" SIMPLY MEANS "SPICE" IN ARABIC. AN ALL-PURPOSE SEASONING IN MIDDLE EASTERN CUISINE, IT IS OFTEN USED AS A RUB ON FISH, POULTRY, AND MEATS OR MIXED WITH OLIVE OIL AND USED AS A VEGETABLE MARINADE. THE COMBINATION OF WARM, SWEET SPICES SUCH AS CINNAMON, CUMIN, CORIANDER, CLOVES, AND PAPRIKA MAKES IT PARTICULARLY AROMATIC. THE ADDITION OF DRIED MINT IS A TURKISH TOUCH.

- ⅓ cup snipped unsulfured dried apricots
- ⅓ cup snipped dried figs
- 1 tablespoon unrefined coconut oil
- 1½ pounds ground chicken breast
- 3 cups sliced leeks (white and light green parts only) (3)
- ⅔ of a medium green and/or red sweet peppers, thinly sliced
- 2 tablespoons Baharat Seasoning (see recipe, below)
- 2 cloves garlic, minced
- 1 cup chopped, seeded tomatoes (2 medium)
- 1 cup chopped, seeded cucumber (½ of a medium)
- ½ cup chopped shelled unsalted pistachios, toasted (see tip)
- ¼ cup snipped fresh mint
- ¼ cup snipped fresh parsley
- 8 to 12 large butterhead or Bibb lettuce leaves

1. Place apricots and figs in a small bowl. Add ⅔ cup boiling water; let stand for 15 minutes. Drain, reserving ½ cup of the liquid.

2. Meanwhile, in an extra-large skillet heat coconut oil over medium heat. Add ground chicken; cook for 3 minutes,

stirring with a wooden spoon to break up meat as it cooks. Add leeks, sweet pepper, Baharat Seasoning, and garlic; cook and stir about 3 minutes or until chicken is done and pepper is just tender. Add apricots, figs, reserved liquid, tomatoes, and cucumber. Cook and stir about 2 minutes or until tomatoes and cucumber just start to break down. Stir in pistachios, mint, and parsley.

3. Serve chicken and vegetables in lettuce leaves.

Baharat Seasoning: In a small bowl combine 2 tablespoons sweet paprika; 1 tablespoon black pepper; 2 teaspoons dried mint, finely crushed; 2 teaspoons ground cumin; 2 teaspoons ground coriander; 2 teaspoons ground cinnamon; 2 teaspoons ground cloves; 1 teaspoon ground nutmeg; and 1 teaspoon ground cardamom. Store in a tightly sealed container at room temperature. Makes about ½ cup.

SPANISH CORNISH HENS

PREP: 10 minutes BAKE: 30 minutes BROIL: 6 minutes MAKES: 2 to 3 servings

THIS RECIPE COULD NOT BE EASIER—AND THE RESULTS ARE ABSOLUTELY AMAZING. COPIOUS AMOUNTS OF SMOKED PAPRIKA, GARLIC, AND LEMON GIVE THESE DIMINUTIVE BIRDS BIG FLAVOR.

2 1½-pound Cornish hens, thawed if frozen
1 tablespoon olive oil
6 cloves garlic, chopped
2 to 3 tablespoons smoked sweet paprika
¼ to ½ teaspoon cayenne pepper (optional)
2 lemons, quartered
2 tablespoons snipped fresh parsley (optional)

1. Preheat oven to 375°F. To quarter the game hens, use kitchen shears or a sharp knife to cut along both sides of the narrow backbone. Butterfly the bird open and cut the hen in half through the breastbone. Remove the hindquarters by cutting through the skin and meat that separates the thighs from the breast. Keep the wing and breast intact. Rub olive oil over Cornish hen pieces. Sprinkle with chopped garlic.

2. Place the hen pieces, skin sides up, in an extra-large oven-going skillet. Sprinkle with smoked paprika and cayenne. Squeeze the lemon quarters over the hens; add lemon quarters to the skillet. Turn hen pieces skin sides down in the pan. Cover and bake for 30 minutes. Remove skillet from oven.

3. Preheat broiler. Using tongs, turn the pieces. Adjust oven rack. Broil 4 to 5 inches from the heat for 6 to 8 minutes until skin is browned and hens are done (175°F). Drizzle with pan juices. If desired, sprinkle with parsley.

PISTACHIO-ROASTED CORNISH HENS WITH ARUGULA, APRICOT, AND FENNEL SALAD

PREP: 30 minutes CHILL: 2 to 12 hours ROAST: 50 minutes STAND: 10 minutes MAKES: 8 servings

A PISTACHIO PESTO MADE WITH PARSLEY, THYME, GARLIC, ORANGE PEEL, ORANGE JUICE, AND OLIVE OIL IS TUCKED UNDER THE SKIN OF EACH BIRD BEFORE MARINATING.

- 4 20- to 24-ounce Cornish game hens
- 3 cups raw pistachio nuts
- 2 tablespoons snipped fresh Italian (flat-leaf) parsley
- 1 tablespoon snipped thyme
- 1 large clove garlic, minced
- 2 teaspoons finely shredded orange peel
- 2 tablespoons fresh orange juice
- ¾ cup olive oil
- 2 large onions, thinly sliced
- ½ cup fresh orange juice
- 2 tablespoons fresh lemon juice
- ¼ teaspoon freshly ground black pepper
- ¼ teaspoon dry mustard
- 2 5-ounce packages arugula
- 1 large bulb fennel, thinly shaved
- 2 tablespoons snipped fennel fronds
- 4 apricots, pitted and cut into thin wedges

1. Rinse inside cavities of Cornish game hens. Tie legs together with 100%-cotton kitchen string. Tuck wings under bodies; set aside.

2. In a food processor or blender combine pistachios, parsley, thyme, garlic, orange peel, and orange juice. Process until coarse paste forms. With processor running, add ¼ cup of the olive oil in a slow, steady stream.

3. Using fingers, loosen skin on the breast side of a hen to make a pocket. Spread one-fourth of the pistachio mixture evenly under the skin. Repeat with remaining hens and pistachio mixture. Spread sliced onions over bottom of roasting pan; place hens, breast sides up, on top of onions. Cover and refrigerate for 2 to 12 hours.

4. Preheat oven to 425°F. Roast hens for 30 to 35 minutes or until an instant-read thermometer inserted in an inside thigh muscle registers 175°F.

5. Meanwhile, for dressing, in a small bowl combine orange juice, lemon juice, pepper, and mustard. Mix well. Add the remaining ½ cup olive oil in a slow steady stream, whisking constantly.

6. For salad, in a large bowl combine arugula, fennel, fennel fronds, and apricots. Drizzle lightly with dressing; toss well. Reserve additional dressing for another purpose.

7. Remove hens from oven; tent loosely with foil and let stand 10 minutes. To serve, divide the salad evenly among eight serving plates. Cut hens in half lengthwise; place hen halves on salads. Serve immediately.

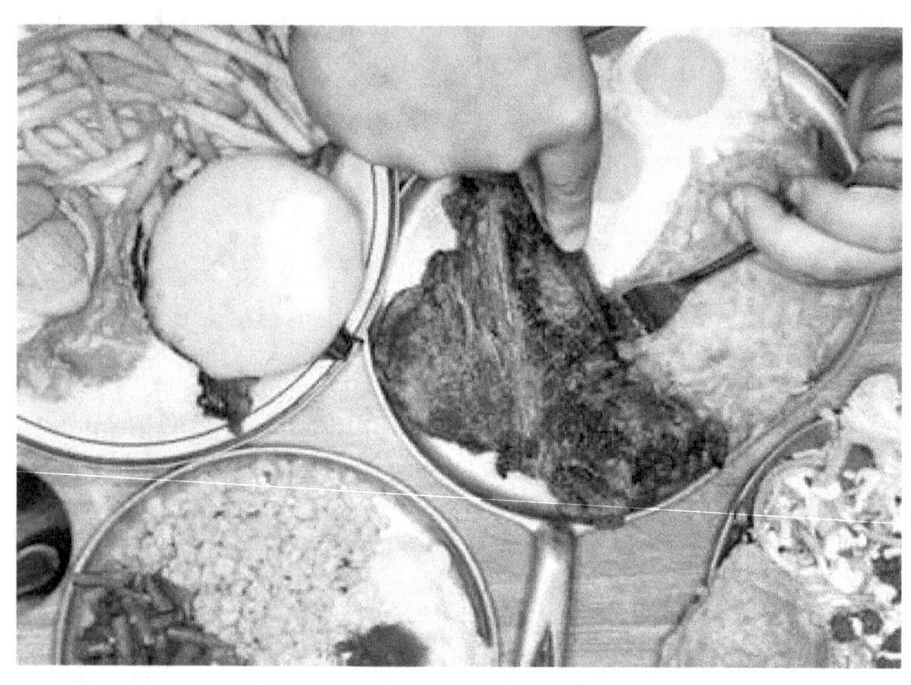

DUCK BREAST WITH POMEGRANATE AND JICAMA SALAD

PREP: 15 minutes COOK: 15 minutes MAKES: 4 servings

CUTTING A DIAMOND PATTERN INTO THE FAT OF THE DUCK BREASTS ALLOWS THE FAT TO RENDER OUT AS THE GARAM MASALA-SEASONED BREASTS COOK. THE DRIPPINGS ARE COMBINED WITH JICAMA, POMEGRANATE SEEDS, ORANGE JUICE, AND BEEF BROTH AND TOSSED WITH PEPPERY GREENS TO WILT THEM JUST SLIGHTLY.

4 boneless Muscovy duck breasts (about 1½ to 2 pounds total)
1 tablespoon garam masala
1 tablespoon unrefined coconut oil
2 cups diced, peeled jicama
½ cup pomegranate seeds
¼ cup fresh orange juice
¼ cup Beef Bone Broth (see recipe) or no-salt-added beef broth
3 cups watercress, stems removed
3 cups torn frisée and/or thinly sliced Belgian endive

1. With a sharp knife, make shallow cuts in diamond patterns into the fat of duck breasts at 1-inch intervals. Sprinkle both sides of the breast halves with the garam masala. Heat an extra-large skillet over medium heat. Melt the coconut oil in the hot skillet. Place breast halves, skin sides down, in the skillet. Cook for 8 minutes with the skin sides down, being careful not to brown too quickly (reduce heat if necessary). Turn duck breasts over; cook for 5 to 6 minutes more or until an instant-read thermometer inserted into breast halves registers 145°F

for medium. Remove breast halves, reserving drippings in a skillet; cover with foil to keep warm.

2. For dressing, add jicama to drippings in skillet; cook and stir for 2 minutes over medium heat. Add pomegranate seeds, orange juice, and Beef Bone Broth to skillet. Bring to boiling; immediately remove from heat.

3. For salad, in a large bowl combine watercress and frisée. Pour hot dressing over greens; toss to coat.

4. Divide salad among four dinner plates. Thinly slice the duck breasts and arrange on salads.

ROASTED TURKEY WITH GARLICKY MASHED ROOTS

PREP: 1 hour ROAST: 2 hours 45 minutes STAND: 15 minutes MAKES: 12 to 14 servings

LOOK FOR A TURKEY THAT HAS NOT BEEN INJECTED WITH A SALT SOLUTION. IF THE LABEL SAYS "ENHANCED" OR "SELF-BASTING," IT LIKELY IS FULL OF SODIUM AND OTHER ADDITIVES.

    1 12- to 14–pound turkey
    2 tablespoons Mediterranean Seasoning (see recipe)
    ¼ cup olive oil
    3 pounds medium carrots, peeled, trimmed, and halved or quartered lengthwise
    1 recipe Garlicky Mashed Roots (see recipe, below)

1. Preheat oven to 425°F. Remove neck and giblets from turkey; reserve for another use if desired. Carefully loosen skin from the edge of the breast. Run your fingers under the skin to create a pocket on top of the breast and on top of the drumsticks. Spoon 1 tablespoon of the Mediterranean Seasoning under the skin; use your fingers to evenly spread it over the breast and drumsticks. Pull neck skin to the back; fasten with a skewer. Tuck ends of drumsticks under the band of skin across the tail. If there is no band of skin, tie drumsticks securely to the tail with 100%-cotton kitchen string. Twist wing tips under the back.

2. Place turkey, breast side up, on a rack in a shallow extra-large roasting pan. Brush turkey with 2 tablespoons of the oil. Sprinkle turkey with remaining Mediterranean Seasoning. Insert an oven-going meat thermometer into

the center of an inside thigh muscle; the thermometer should not touch bone. Cover turkey loosely with foil.

3. Roast for 30 minutes. Reduce oven temperature to 325°F. Roast for 1½ hours. In an extra-large bowl combine carrots and the remaining 2 tablespoons oil; toss to coat. Spread carrots in a large rimmed baking pan. Remove foil from turkey and cut band of skin or string between drumsticks. Roast carrots and turkey for 45 minutes to 1¼ hours more or until the thermometer registers 175°F.

4. Remove turkey from oven. Cover; let stand for 15 to 20 minutes before carving. Serve turkey with carrots and Garlicky Mashed Roots.

Garlicky Mashed Roots: Trim and peel 3 to 3½ pounds rutabagas and 1½ to 2 pounds celery root; cut into 2-inch pieces. In a 6-quart pot cook rutabagas and celery root in enough boiling water to cover for 25 to 30 minutes or until very tender. Meanwhile, in a small saucepan combine 3 tablespoons extra virgin oil and 6 to 8 cloves minced garlic. Cook over low heat for 5 to 10 minutes or until garlic is very fragrant but not browned. Carefully add ¾ cup Chicken Bone Broth (see recipe) or no-salt-added chicken broth. Bring to boiling; remove from heat. Drain vegetables and return to the pot. Mash vegetables with a potato masher or beat with an electric mixer on low. Add ½ teaspoon black pepper. Gradually mash or beat in broth mixture until vegetables are combined and nearly smooth. If necessary, add an additional ¼ cup Chicken Bone Broth to make desired consistency.

STUFFED TURKEY BREAST WITH PESTO SAUCE AND ARUGULA SALAD

PREP: 30 minutes ROAST: 1 hour 30 minutes STAND: 20 minutes MAKES: 6 servings

THIS IS FOR THE WHITE-MEAT LOVERS OUT THERE—A CRISP-SKINNED BREAST OF TURKEY STUFFED WITH DRIED TOMATOES, BASIL, AND MEDITERRANEAN SPICES. LEFTOVERS MAKE A GREAT LUNCH.

- 1 cup unsulfured dried tomatoes (not oil-packed)
- 1 4-pound boneless turkey breast half with skin
- 3 teaspoons Mediterranean Seasoning (see recipe)
- 1 cup loosely packed fresh basil leaves
- 1 tablespoon olive oil
- 8 ounces baby arugula
- 3 large tomatoes, halved and sliced
- ¼ cup olive oil
- 2 tablespoons red wine vinegar
- Black pepper
- 1½ cups Basil Pesto (see recipe)

1. Preheat oven to 375°F. In a small bowl pour enough boiling water over dried tomatoes to cover. Let stand for 5 minutes; drain and finely chop.

2. Place turkey breast, skin side down, on a large sheet of plastic wrap. Place another sheet of plastic wrap over turkey. Using the flat side of a meat mallet, gently pound breast to an even thickness, about ¾ inch thick. Discard plastic wrap. Sprinkle 1½ teaspoons of the Mediterranean Seasoning over the meat. Top with the tomatoes and basil leaves. Carefully roll up turkey breast, keeping skin on the

outside. Using 100%-cotton kitchen string, tie roast in four to six places to secure. Brush with 1 tablespoon olive oil. Sprinkle roast with the remaining 1½ teaspoons Mediterranean Seasoning.

3. Place roast on a rack set in a shallow pan with the skin side up. Roast, uncovered, for 1½ hours or until an instant-read thermometer inserted near the center registers 165°F and skin is golden brown and crisp. Remove turkey from oven. Cover loosely with foil; let stand for 20 minutes before slicing.

4. For arugula salad, in a large bowl combine arugula, tomatoes, ¼ cup olive oil, the vinegar, and pepper to taste. Remove strings from roast. Thinly slice turkey. Serve with arugula salad and Basil Pesto.

SPICED TURKEY BREAST WITH CHERRY BBQ SAUCE

PREP: 15 minutes ROAST: 1 hour 15 minutes STAND: 45 minutes MAKES: 6 to 8 servings

THIS IS A NICE RECIPE FOR SERVING A CROWD AT A BACKYARD BARBECUE WHEN YOU WANT TO DO SOMETHING OTHER THAN BURGERS. SERVE IT WITH A CRISP SALAD, SUCH AS CRUNCHY BROCCOLI SALAD (SEE <u>RECIPE</u>) OR SHAVED BRUSSELS SPROUTS SALAD (SEE <u>RECIPE</u>).

- 1 4- to 5-pound whole bone-in turkey breast
- 3 tablespoons Smoky Seasoning (see <u>recipe</u>)
- 2 tablespoons fresh lemon juice
- 3 tablespoons olive oil
- 1 cup dry white wine, such as Sauvignon Blanc
- 1 cup fresh or frozen unsweetened Bing cherries, pitted and chopped
- ⅓ cup water
- 1 cup BBQ Sauce (see <u>recipe</u>)

1. Let turkey breast stand at room temperature for 30 minutes. Preheat oven to 325°F. Place the turkey breast, skin side up, on a rack in a roasting pan.

2. In a small bowl combine the Smoky Seasoning, lemon juice, and olive oil to make a paste. Loosen the skin from the meat; gently spread half of the paste onto the meat under the skin. Spread the remaining paste evenly over the skin. Pour the wine into the bottom of the roasting pan.

3. Roast for 1¼ to 1½ hours or until the skin is golden brown and an instant-read thermometer inserted into center of roast (not touching bone) registers 170°F, turning the

roasting pan halfway through cooking time. Let stand for 15 to 30 minutes before carving.

4. Meanwhile, for Cherry BBQ Sauce, in a medium saucepan combine cherries and the water. Bring to boiling; reduce heat. Simmer, uncovered, for 5 minutes. Stir in BBQ Sauce; simmer for 5 minutes. Serve warm or at room temperature with the turkey.

WINE-BRAISED TURKEY TENDERLOIN

PREP: 30 minutes COOK: 35 minutes MAKES: 4 servings

COOKING THE PAN-SEARED TURKEY IN A COMBINATION OF WINE, CHOPPED ROMA TOMATOES, CHICKEN BROTH, FRESH HERBS, AND CRUSHED RED PEPPER INFUSES IT WITH GREAT FLAVOR. SERVE THIS STEWLIKE DISH IN SHALLOW BOWLS AND WITH BIG SPOONS TO GET SOME OF THE TASTY BROTH WITH EVERY BITE.

2 8- to 12-ounce turkey tenderloins, cut into 1-inch pieces
2 tablespoons no-salt-added poultry seasoning
2 tablespoons olive oil
6 cloves garlic, minced (1 tablespoon)
1 cup chopped onion
½ cup chopped celery
6 roma tomatoes, seeded and chopped (about 3 cups)
½ cup dry white wine, such as Sauvignon Blanc
½ cup Chicken Bone Broth (see recipe) or no-salt-added chicken broth
½ teaspoon finely snipped fresh rosemary
¼ to ½ teaspoon crushed red pepper
½ cup fresh basil leaves, chopped
½ cup snipped fresh parsley

1. In a large bowl toss turkey pieces with poultry seasoning to coat. In an extra-large nonstick skillet heat 1 tablespoon of the olive oil over medium heat. Cook turkey in batches in hot oil until browned on all sides. (Turkey does not need to be cooked through.) Transfer to a plate and keep warm.

2. Add the remaining 1 tablespoon olive oil to the pan. Increase heat to medium-high. Add the garlic; cook and stir for 1 minute. Add onion and celery; cook and stir for 5

minutes. Add the turkey and any juices from the plate, tomatoes, wine, Chicken Bone Broth, rosemary, and crushed red pepper. Reduce heat to medium-low. Cover and cook for 20 minutes, stirring occasionally. Add basil and parsley. Uncover and cook for 5 minutes more or until turkey is no longer pink.

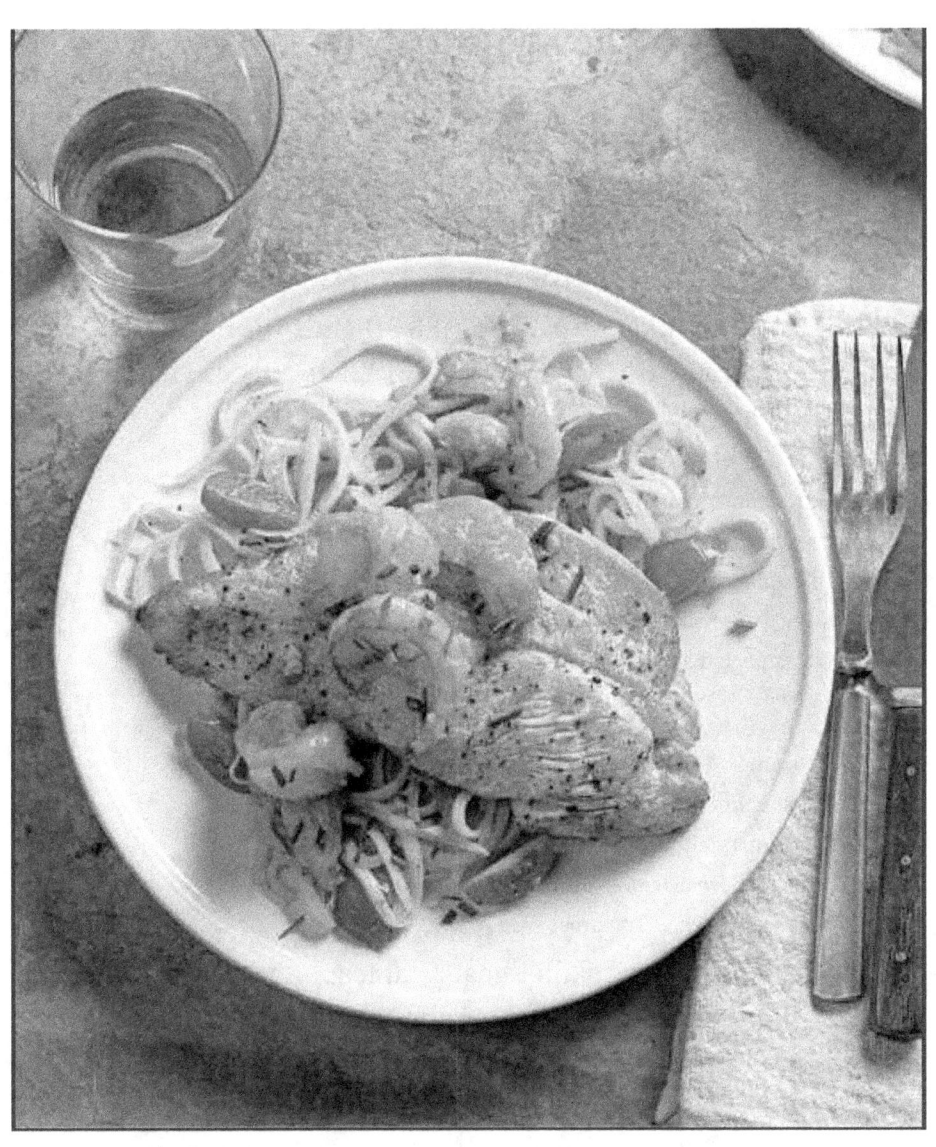

PAN-SAUTÉED TURKEY BREAST WITH CHIVE SCAMPI SAUCE

PREP: 30 minutes COOK: 15 minutes MAKES: 4 servings PHOTO

TO CUT THE TURKEY TENDERLOINS IN HALF HORIZONTALLY AS EVENLY AS POSSIBLE, LIGHTLY PRESS DOWN ON EACH ONE WITH THE PALM OF YOUR HAND, APPLYING CONSISTENT PRESSURE, AS YOU CUT THROUGH THE MEAT.

¼ cup olive oil

2 8- to 12-ounce turkey breast tenderloins, cut in half horizontally

¼ teaspoon freshly ground black pepper

3 tablespoons olive oil

4 cloves garlic, minced

8 ounces peeled and deveined medium shrimp, tails removed and halved lengthwise

¼ cup dry white wine, Chicken Bone Broth (see recipe), or no-salt-added chicken broth

2 tablespoons snipped fresh chives

½ teaspoon finely shredded lemon peel

1 tablespoon fresh lemon juice

Squash Noodles and Tomatoes (see recipe, below) (optional)

1. In an extra-large skillet heat 1 tablespoon of the olive oil over medium-high heat. Add turkey to skillet; sprinkle with pepper. Reduce heat to medium. Cook for 12 to 15 minutes or until no longer pink and juices run clear (165°F), turning once halfway through cooking time. Remove turkey steaks from skillet. Cover with foil to keep warm.

2. For sauce, in the same skillet heat the 3 tablespoons oil over medium heat. Add garlic; cook for 30 seconds. Stir in

shrimp; cook and stir for 1 minute. Stir in wine, chives, and lemon peel; cook and stir for 1 minute more or until shrimp are opaque. Remove from heat; stir in lemon juice. To serve, spoon sauce over turkey steaks. If desired, serve with Squash Noodles and Tomatoes.

Squash Noodles and Tomatoes: Using a mandoline or julienne peeler, slice 2 yellow summer squash into julienne strips. In a large skillet heat 1 tablespoon extra virgin olive oil over medium-high heat. Add squash strips; cook for 2 minutes. Add 1 cup quartered grape tomatoes and ¼ teaspoon freshly ground black pepper; cook for 2 minutes more or until squash is crisp-tender.

BRAISED TURKEY LEGS WITH ROOT VEGETABLES

PREP: 30 minutes COOK: 1 hour 45 minutes MAKES: 4 servings

THIS IS ONE OF THOSE DISHES YOU WANT TO MAKE ON A CRISP FALL AFTERNOON WHEN YOU HAVE TIME TO TAKE A WALK WHILE IT SIMMERS IN THE OVEN. IF THE EXERCISE DOESN'T STIR UP AN APPETITE, THE WONDERFUL AROMA WHEN YOU WALK THROUGH THE DOOR CERTAINLY WILL.

3 tablespoons olive oil
4 20- to 24-ounce turkey legs
½ teaspoon freshly ground black pepper
6 cloves garlic, peeled and crushed
1½ teaspoons fennel seeds, bruised
1 teaspoon whole allspice, bruised*
1½ cups Chicken Bone Broth (see recipe) or no-salt-added chicken broth
2 sprigs fresh rosemary
2 sprigs fresh thyme
1 bay leaf
2 large onions, peeled and cut into 8 wedges each
6 large carrots, peeled and cut into 1-inch slices
2 large turnips, peeled and cut into 1-inch cubes
2 medium parsnips, peeled and cut into 1-inch slices**
1 celery root, peeled and cut into 1-inch pieces

1. Preheat oven to 350°F. In a large skillet heat the olive oil over medium-high heat until shimmering. Add 2 of the turkey legs. Cook about 8 minutes or until legs are golden brown and crisp on all sides, turning to brown evenly. Transfer turkey legs to a plate; repeat with remaining 2 turkey legs. Set aside.

2. Add pepper, garlic, fennel seeds, and allspice seeds to the skillet. Cook and stir over medium heat for 1 to 2 minutes or until fragrant. Stir in Chicken Bone Broth, rosemary, thyme, and bay leaf. Bring to boiling, stirring to scrape browned bits from the bottom of the skillet. Remove skillet from heat and set aside.

3. In an extra-large Dutch oven with a tight-fitting lid combine onions, carrots, turnips, parsnips, and celery root. Add liquid from skillet; toss to coat. Press turkey legs into the vegetable mixture. Cover with lid.

4. Bake about 1 hour 45 minutes or until vegetables are tender and turkey is cooked through. Serve turkey legs and vegetables in large shallow bowls. Drizzle juices from pan over top.

*Tip: To bruise allspice and fennel seeds, place seeds on a cutting board. Using a flat side of a chef's knife, press down to lightly crush the seeds.

**Tip: Cube any large pieces from the tops of the parsnips.

HERBED TURKEY MEAT LOAF WITH CARAMELIZED ONION KETCHUP AND ROASTED CABBAGE WEDGES

PREP: 15 minutes COOK: 30 minutes BAKE: 1 hour 10 minutes STAND: 5 minutes
MAKES: 4 servings

CLASSIC KETCHUP-TOPPED MEAT LOAF IS DEFINITELY ON THE PALEO MENU WHEN THE KETCHUP (SEE RECIPE) IS FREE OF SALT AND ADDED SUGARS. HERE THE KETCHUP IS STIRRED TOGETHER WITH CARAMELIZED ONIONS, WHICH ARE PILED ON TOP OF THE MEAT LOAF BEFORE BAKING.

- 1½ pounds ground turkey
- 2 eggs, lightly beaten
- ½ cup almond meal
- ⅓ cup snipped fresh parsley
- ¼ cup thinly sliced scallions (2)
- 1 tablespoon snipped fresh sage or 1 teaspoon dried sage, crushed
- 1 tablespoon snipped fresh thyme or 1 teaspoon dried thyme, crushed
- ¼ teaspoon black pepper
- 2 tablespoons olive oil
- 2 sweet onions, halved and thinly sliced
- 1 cup Paleo Ketchup (see recipe)
- 1 small head cabbage, halved, cored, and cut into 8 wedges
- ½ to 1 teaspoon crushed red pepper

1. Preheat oven to 350°F. Line a large roasting pan with parchment paper; set aside. In a large bowl combine ground turkey, eggs, almond meal, parsley, scallions, sage, thyme, and black pepper. In the prepared roasting pan shape turkey mixture into an 8×4-inch loaf. Bake for 30 minutes.

2. Meanwhile, for the caramelized onion ketchup, in a large skillet heat 1 tablespoon of the olive oil over medium heat. Add onions; cook about 5 minutes or until onions just start to brown, stirring frequently. Reduce heat to medium-low; cook about 25 minutes or until golden and very soft, stirring occasionally. Remove from heat; stir in Paleo Ketchup.

3. Spoon some of the caramelized onion ketchup over turkey loaf. Arrange cabbage wedges around loaf. Drizzle cabbage with the remaining 1 tablespoon olive oil; sprinkle with crushed red pepper. Bake about 40 minutes or until an instant-read thermometer inserted in center of loaf registers 165°F, topping with additional caramelized onion ketchup and turning the cabbage wedges after 20 minutes. Let turkey loaf stand for 5 to 10 minutes before slicing.

4. Serve turkey loaf with cabbage wedges and any remaining caramelized onion ketchup.

TURKEY POSOLE

PREP: 20 minutes BROIL: 8 minutes COOK: 16 minutes MAKES: 4 servings

THE TOPPINGS ON THIS WARMING, MEXICAN-STYLE SOUP ARE MORE THAN GARNISHES. THE CILANTRO ADDS DISTINCTIVE FLAVOR, AVOCADO CONTRIBUTES CREAMINESS—AND TOASTED PEPITAS PROVIDE A DELIGHTFUL CRUNCH.

8 fresh tomatillos
1¼ to 1½ pounds ground turkey
1 red sweet pepper, seeded and cut into thin bite-size strips
½ cup chopped onion (1 medium)
6 cloves garlic, minced (1 tablespoon)
1 tablespoon Mexican Seasoning (see recipe)
2 cups Chicken Bone Broth (see recipe) or no-salt-added chicken broth
1 14.5-ounce can no-salt-added fire-roasted tomatoes, undrained
1 jalapeño or serrano chile pepper, seeded and minced (see tip)
1 medium avocado, halved, peeled, seeded, and thinly sliced
¼ cup unsalted pepitas, toasted (see tip)
¼ cup snipped fresh cilantro
Lime wedges

1. Preheat the broiler. Remove husks from tomatillos and discard. Wash tomatillos and cut into halves. Place tomatillo halves on the unheated rack of a broiler pan. Broil 4 to 5 inches from the heat for 8 to 10 minutes or until lightly charred, turning once halfway through broiling. Cool slightly on pan on a wire rack.

2. Meanwhile, in a large skillet cook turkey, sweet pepper, and onion over medium-high heat for 5 to 10 minutes or until turkey is browned and vegetables are tender, stirring with a wooden spoon to break up meat as it cooks. Drain off fat

if necessary. Add garlic and Mexican Seasoning. Cook and stir for 1 minute more.

3. In a blender combine about two-thirds of the charred tomatillos and 1 cup of the Chicken Bone Broth. Cover and blend until smooth. Add to turkey mixture in skillet. Stir in the remaining 1 cup Chicken Bone Broth, undrained tomatoes, and chile pepper. Coarsely chop the remaining tomatillos; add to the turkey mixture. Bring to boiling; reduce heat. Cover and simmer for 10 minutes.

4. To serve, ladle soup into shallow serving bowls. Top with avocado, pepitas, and cilantro. Pass lime wedges to squeeze over soup.

CHICKEN BONE BROTH

PREP: 15 minutes ROAST: 30 minutes COOK: 4 hours CHILL: overnight MAKES: about 10 cups

FOR THE FRESHEST, BEST TASTE—AND HIGHEST NUTRIENT CONTENT—USE HOMEMADE CHICKEN BROTH IN YOUR RECIPES. (IT ALSO DOESN'T CONTAIN ANY SALT, PRESERVATIVES, OR ADDITIVES.) ROASTING THE BONES BEFORE SIMMERING ENHANCES FLAVOR. AS THEY SLOWLY COOK IN LIQUID, THE BONES INFUSE THE BROTH WITH MINERALS SUCH AS CALCIUM, PHOSPHORUS, MAGNESIUM, AND POTASSIUM. THE SLOW COOKER VARIATION BELOW MAKES IT ESPECIALLY EASY TO DO. FREEZE IT IN 2- AND 4-CUP CONTAINERS AND THAW ONLY WHAT YOU NEED.

- 2 pounds chicken wings and backs
- 4 carrots, chopped
- 2 large leeks, white and pale green parts only, thinly sliced
- 2 stalks celery with leaves, coarsely chopped
- 1 parsnip, coarsely chopped
- 6 large sprigs Italian (flat-leaf) parsley
- 6 sprigs fresh thyme
- 4 cloves garlic, halved
- 2 teaspoons whole black peppercorns
- 2 whole cloves
- Cold water

1. Preheat oven to 425°F. Arrange chicken wings and backs on a large baking sheet; roast for 30 to 35 minutes or until well browned.

2. Transfer browned chicken pieces and any browned bits accumulated on the baking sheet to a large stockpot. Add

carrots, leeks, celery, parsnip, parsley, thyme, garlic, peppercorns, and cloves. Add enough cold water (about 12 cups) to a large stockpot to cover chicken and vegetables. Bring to simmering over medium heat; adjust heat to maintain broth at a very low simmer, with bubbles just breaking the surface. Cover and simmer for 4 hours.

3. Strain hot broth through a large colander lined with two layers of damp 100%-cotton cheesecloth. Discard solids. Cover broth and chill overnight. Before using, remove fat layer from top of broth and discard.

Tip: To clarify stock (optional), in a small bowl combine 1 egg white, 1 crushed eggshell, and ¼ cup cold water. Stir mixture into strained stock in pot. Return to boiling. Remove from heat; let stand for 5 minutes. Strain hot broth through a colander lined with a fresh double layer of 100%-cotton cheesecloth. Chill and skim fat before using.

Slow Cooker Directions: Prepare as directed, except in Step 2 place ingredients in a 5- to 6-quart slow cooker. Cover and cook on low-heat setting for 12 to 14 hours. Continue as directed in Step 3. Makes about 10 cups.

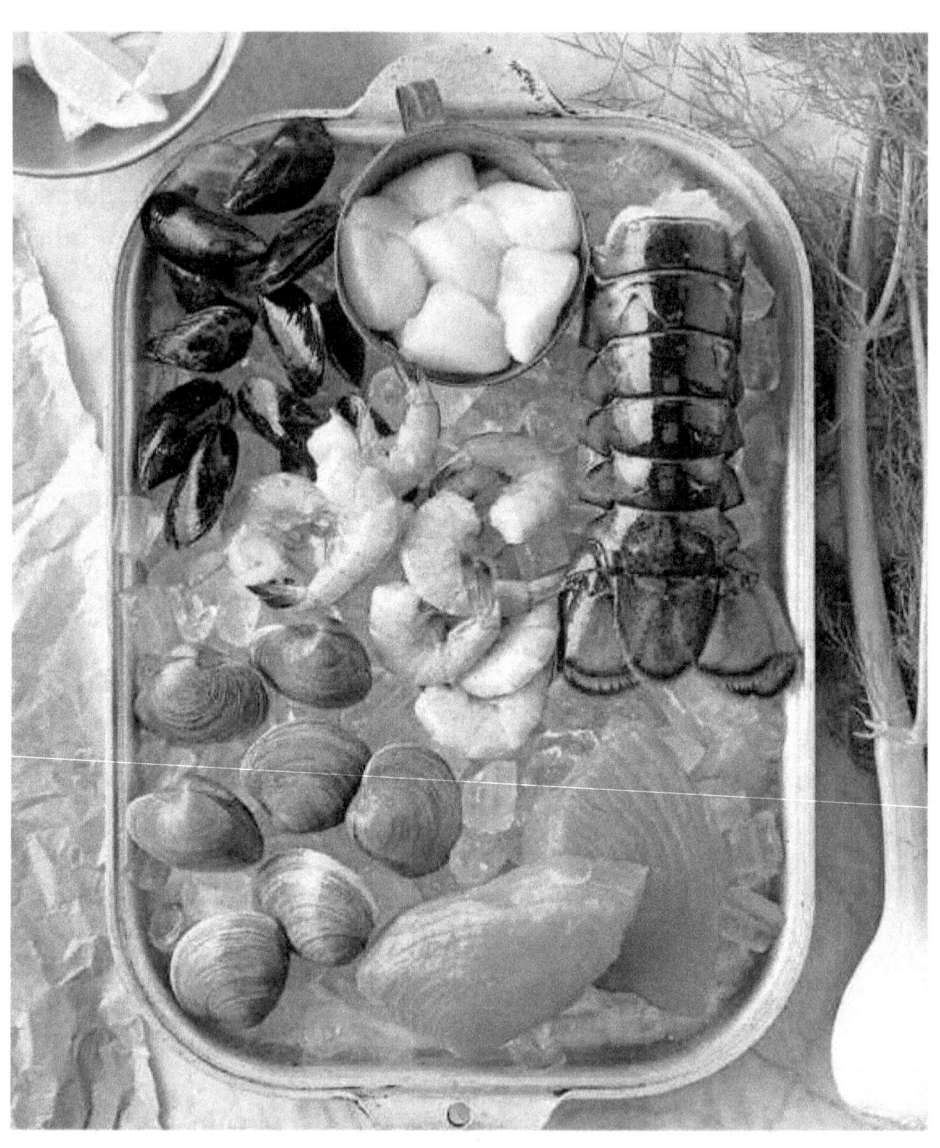

GREEN HARISSA SALMON

PREP: 25 minutes BAKE: 10 minutes GRILL: 8 minutes MAKES: 4 servings PHOTO

A STANDARD VEGETABLE PEELER IS USED TO SHAVE FRESH RAW ASPARAGUS INTO THIN RIBBONS FOR THE SALAD. TOSSED WITH BRIGHT CITRUS VINAIGRETTE (SEE RECIPE) AND TOPPED WITH SMOKY TOASTED SUNFLOWER SEEDS, IT'S A REFRESHING ACCOMPANIMENT TO THE SALMON AND SPICY GREEN HERB SAUCE.

SALMON
- 4 6- to 8-ounce fresh or frozen skinless salmon fillets, about 1 inch thick
- Olive oil

HARISSA
- 1½ teaspoons cumin seeds
- 1½ teaspoons coriander seeds
- 1 cup tightly packed fresh parsley leaves
- 1 cup roughly chopped fresh cilantro (leaves and stems)
- 2 jalapeños, seeded and coarsely chopped (see tip)
- 1 scallion, cut up
- 2 cloves garlic
- 1 teaspoon finely shredded lemon peel
- 2 tablespoons fresh lemon juice
- ⅓ cup olive oil

SPICED SUNFLOWER SEEDS
- ⅓ cup raw sunflower seeds
- 1 teaspoon olive oil
- 1 teaspoon Smoky Seasoning (see recipe)

SALAD
- 12 large asparagus spears, trimmed (about 1 pound)
- ⅓ cup Bright Citrus Vinaigrette (see recipe)

1. Thaw fish, if frozen; pat dry with paper towels. Brush both sides of fish lightly with olive oil. Set aside.

2. For harissa, in a small skillet toast cumin seeds and coriander seeds over medium-low heat for 3 to 4 minutes or until lightly toasted and fragrant. In a food processor combine toasted cumin and coriander seeds, the parsley, cilantro, jalapeños, scallion, garlic, lemon peel, lemon juice, and olive oil. Process until smooth. Set aside.

3. For spiced sunflower seeds, preheat oven to 300°F. Line a baking sheet with parchment paper; set aside. In a small bowl combine sunflower seeds and 1 teaspoon olive oil. Sprinkle the Smoky Seasoning over the seeds; stir to coat. Spread sunflower seeds evenly on the parchment paper. Bake about 10 minutes or until lightly toasted.

4. For a charcoal or gas grill, place salmon on a greased grill rack directly over medium heat. Cover and grill for 8 to 12 minutes or until fish begins to flake when tested with a fork, turning once halfway through grilling.

5. Meanwhile, for salad, using a vegetable peeler, shave asparagus spears into long thin ribbons. Transfer to a platter or medium bowl. (The tips will snap off as the spears get thinner; add them to platter or bowl.) Drizzle the Bright Citrus Vinaigrette over shaved spears. Sprinkle with spiced sunflower seeds.

6. To serve, place a fillet on each of four plates; spoon some of the green harissa on each fillet. Serve with shaved asparagus salad.

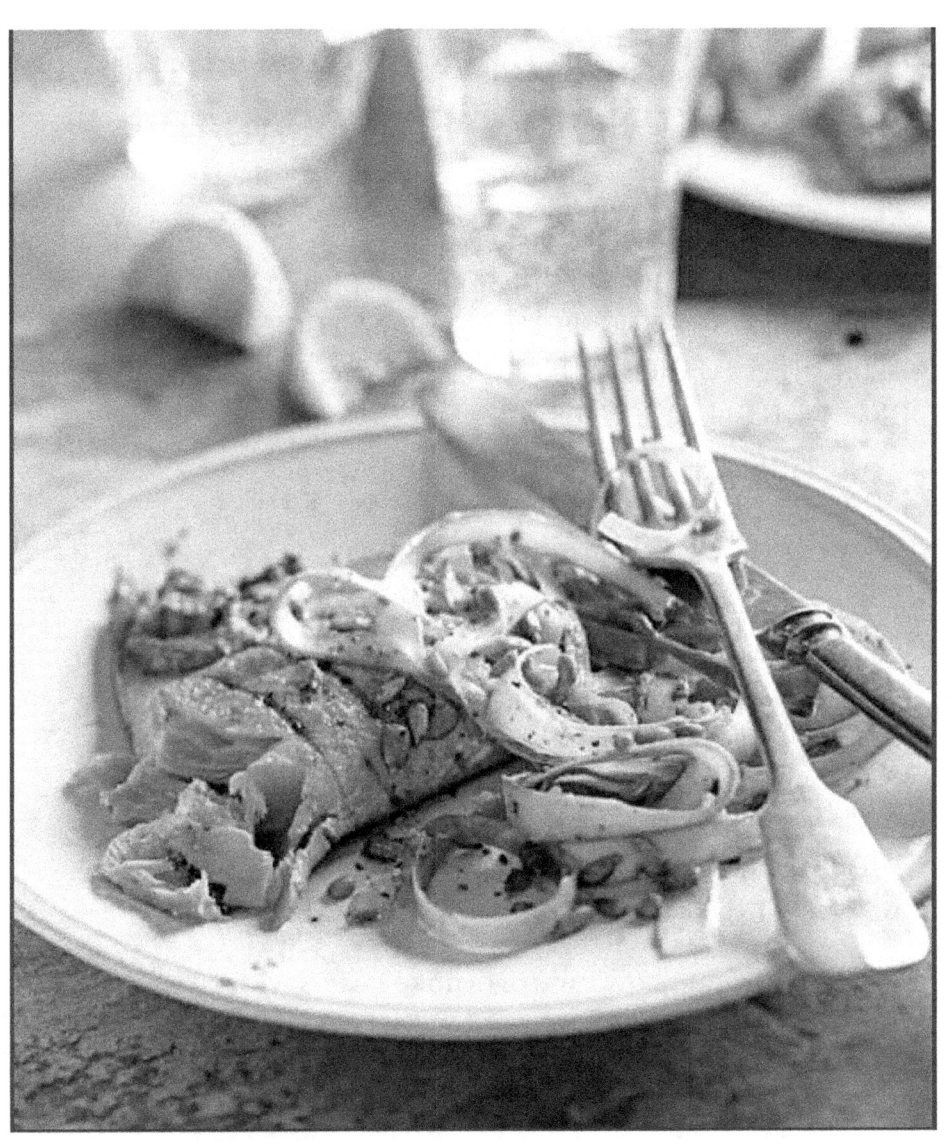

GRILLED SALMON WITH MARINATED ARTICHOKE HEART SALAD

PREP: 20 minutes GRILL: 12 minutes MAKES: 4 servings

OFTENTIMES, THE BEST TOOLS FOR TOSSING A SALAD ARE YOUR HANDS. GETTING THE TENDER LETTUCES AND GRILLED ARTICHOKES TO INCORPORATE EVENLY IN THIS SALAD IS BEST DONE WITH CLEAN HANDS.

- 4 6-ounce fresh or frozen salmon fillets
- 1 9-ounce package frozen artichoke hearts, thawed and drained
- 5 tablespoons olive oil
- 2 tablespoons minced shallots
- 1 tablespoon finely shredded lemon peel
- ¼ cup fresh lemon juice
- 3 tablespoons snipped fresh oregano
- ½ teaspoon freshly ground black pepper
- 1 tablespoon Mediterranean Seasoning (see recipe)
- 1 5-ounce package mixed baby lettuces

1. Thaw fish, if frozen. Rinse fish; pat dry with paper towels. Set fish aside.

2. In a medium bowl toss artichoke hearts with 2 tablespoons of the olive oil; set aside. In a large bowl combine 2 tablespoons of the olive oil, the shallots, lemon peel, lemon juice, and oregano; set aside.

3. For a charcoal or gas grill, place the artichoke hearts in a grill basket and grill directly over medium-high heat. Cover and grill for 6 to 8 minutes or until nicely charred and heated through, stirring frequently. Remove artichokes from grill. Let cool 5 minutes, then add

artichokes to shallot mixture. Season with pepper; toss to coat. Set aside.

4. Brush salmon with the remaining 1 tablespoon olive oil; sprinkle with the Mediterranean Seasoning. Place salmon on the grill rack, seasoned sides down, directly over medium-high heat. Cover and grill for 6 to 8 minutes or until fish begins to flake when tested with a fork, carefully turning once halfway through grilling.

5. Add lettuces to bowl with marinated artichokes; toss gently to coat. Serve salad with grilled salmon.

FLASH-ROASTED CHILE-SAGE SALMON WITH GREEN TOMATO SALSA

PREP: 35 minutes CHILL: 2 to 4 hours ROAST: 10 minutes MAKES: 4 servings

"FLASH-ROASTING" REFERS TO THE TECHNIQUE OF HEATING A DRY SKILLET IN THE OVEN AT A HIGH TEMPERATURE, ADDING SOME OIL AND THE FISH, CHICKEN, OR MEAT (IT SIZZLES!), THEN FINISHING THE DISH IN THE OVEN. FLASH-ROASTING CUTS DOWN ON COOKING TIME AND CREATES A DELICIOUSLY CRISP CRUST ON THE EXTERIOR—AND A JUICY, FLAVORFUL INTERIOR.

SALMON

- 4 5- to 6-ounce fresh or frozen salmon fillets
- 3 tablespoons olive oil
- ¼ cup finely chopped onion
- 2 cloves garlic, peeled and sliced
- 1 tablespoon ground coriander
- 1 teaspoon ground cumin
- 2 teaspoons sweet paprika
- 1 teaspoon dried oregano, crushed
- ¼ teaspoon cayenne pepper
- ⅓ cup fresh lime juice
- 1 tablespoon snipped fresh sage

GREEN TOMATO SALSA

- 1½ cups diced firm green tomatoes
- ⅓ cup finely chopped red onion
- 2 tablespoons snipped fresh cilantro
- 1 jalapeño, seeded and minced (see tip)
- 1 clove garlic, minced
- ½ teaspoon ground cumin

¼ teaspoon chili powder

2 to 3 tablespoons fresh lime juice

1. Thaw fish, if frozen. Rinse fish; pat dry with paper towels. Set fish aside.

2. For chile-sage paste, in a small saucepan combine 1 tablespoon of the olive oil, onion, and garlic. Cook over low heat for 1 to 2 minutes or until fragrant. Stir in coriander and cumin; cook and stir for 1 minute. Stir in paprika, oregano, and cayenne pepper; cook and stir for 1 minute. Add lime juice and sage; cook and stir about 3 minutes or just until a smooth paste forms; cool.

3. Using your fingers, coat both sides of fillets with chile-sage paste. Place fish in a glass or nonreactive dish; cover tightly with plastic wrap. Refrigerate for 2 to 4 hours.

4. Meanwhile, for salsa, in a medium bowl combine tomatoes, onion, cilantro, jalapeño, garlic, cumin, and chili powder. Toss well to mix. Drizzle with lime juice; toss to coat.

4. Using a rubber spatula, scrape as much paste as you can off of the salmon. Discard paste.

5. Place an extra-large cast-iron skillet in the oven. Turn oven to 500°F. Preheat oven with skillet in it.

6. Remove hot skillet from oven. Pour 1 tablespoon olive oil into the pan. Tip pan to cover the bottom of the skillet with oil. Place fillets in the skillet, skin sides down. Brush tops of fillets with the remaining 1 tablespoon olive oil.

7. Roast salmon about 10 minutes or until fish begins to flake when tested with a fork. Serve fish with salsa.

ROASTED SALMON AND ASPARAGUS EN PAPILLOTE WITH LEMON-HAZELNUT PESTO

PREP: 20 minutes ROAST: 17 minutes MAKES: 4 servings

COOKING "EN PAPILLOTE" SIMPLY MEANS COOKING IN PAPER. IT IS A BEAUTIFUL WAY TO COOK FOR MANY REASONS. THE FISH AND VEGETABLES STEAM INSIDE THE PARCHMENT PACKET, SEALING IN JUICES, FLAVOR, AND NUTRIENTS—AND THERE ARE NO POTS AND PANS TO WASH AFTERWARDS.

- 4 6-ounce fresh or frozen salmon fillets
- 1 cup lightly packed fresh basil leaves
- 1 cup lightly packed fresh parsley leaves
- ½ cup hazelnuts, toasted*
- 5 tablespoons olive oil
- 1 teaspoon finely shredded lemon peel
- 2 tablespoons fresh lemon juice
- 1 clove garlic, chopped
- 1 pound slender asparagus, trimmed
- 4 tablespoons dry white wine

1. Thaw salmon, if frozen. Rinse fish; pat dry with paper towels. Preheat oven to 400°F.

2. For pesto, in a blender or food processor combine basil, parsley, hazelnuts, olive oil, lemon peel, lemon juice, and garlic. Cover and blend or process until smooth; set aside.

3. Cut four 12-inch squares of parchment paper. For each packet, place a salmon fillet in the center of a parchment square. Top with one-fourth of the asparagus and 2 to 3

tablespoons pesto; drizzle with 1 tablespoon wine. Bring up two opposite sides of the parchment paper and fold together several times over fish. Fold ends of parchment to seal. Repeat to make three more packets.

4. Roast for 17 to 19 minutes or until fish begins to flake when tested with a fork (carefully open packet to check doneness).

*Tip: To toast hazelnuts, preheat oven to 350°F. Spread nuts in a single layer in a shallow baking pan. Bake for 8 to 10 minutes or until lightly toasted, stirring once to toast evenly. Cool nuts slightly. Place warm nuts on a clean kitchen towel; rub with the towel to remove the loose skins.

SPICE-RUBBED SALMON WITH MUSHROOM-APPLE PAN SAUCE

START TO FINISH: 40 minutes MAKES: 4 servings

THIS WHOLE SALMON FILLET TOPPED WITH A MIXTURE OF SAUTÉED MUSHROOMS, SHALLOT, RED-SKINNED APPLE SLICES—AND SERVED ON A BED OF BRIGHT-GREEN SPINACH—MAKES AN IMPRESSIVE DISH TO SERVE TO GUESTS.

- 1 1½-pound fresh or frozen whole salmon fillet, skin on
- 1 teaspoon fennel seeds, finely crushed*
- ½ teaspoon dried sage, crushed
- ½ teaspoon ground coriander
- ¼ teaspoon dry mustard
- ¼ teaspoon black pepper
- 2 tablespoons olive oil
- 1½ cups fresh cremini mushrooms, quartered
- 1 medium shallot, very thinly sliced
- 1 small cooking apple, quartered, cored, and thinly sliced
- ¼ cup dry white wine
- 4 cups fresh spinach
- Small sprigs fresh sage (optional)

1. Thaw salmon, if frozen. Preheat oven to 425°F. Line a large baking sheet with parchment paper; set aside. Rinse fish; pat dry with paper towels. Place salmon, skin side down, on prepared baking sheet. In a small bowl combine fennel seeds, ½ teaspoon dried sage, coriander, mustard, and pepper. Sprinkle evenly over salmon; rub in with your fingers.

2. Measure thickness of fish. Roast salmon for 4 to 6 minutes per ½-inch thickness or until fish begins to flake when tested with a fork.

3. Meanwhile, for pan sauce, in a large skillet heat olive oil over medium heat. Add mushrooms and shallot; cook for 6 to 8 minutes or until mushrooms are tender and starting to brown, stirring occasionally. Add apple; cover and cook and stir for 4 minutes more. Carefully add wine. Cook, uncovered, for 2 to 3 minutes or until apple slices are just tender. Using a slotted spoon, transfer mushroom mixture to a medium bowl; cover to keep warm.

4. In the same skillet cook spinach for 1 minute or until spinach is just wilted, stirring constantly. Divide spinach among four serving plates. Cut salmon fillet into four equal portions, cutting to, but not through, the skin. Use a large spatula to lift salmon portions off of the skin; place one salmon portion on spinach on each plate. Spoon mushroom mixture evenly over salmon. If desired, garnish with fresh sage.

*Tip: Use a mortar and pestle or spice grinder to finely crush the fennel seeds.

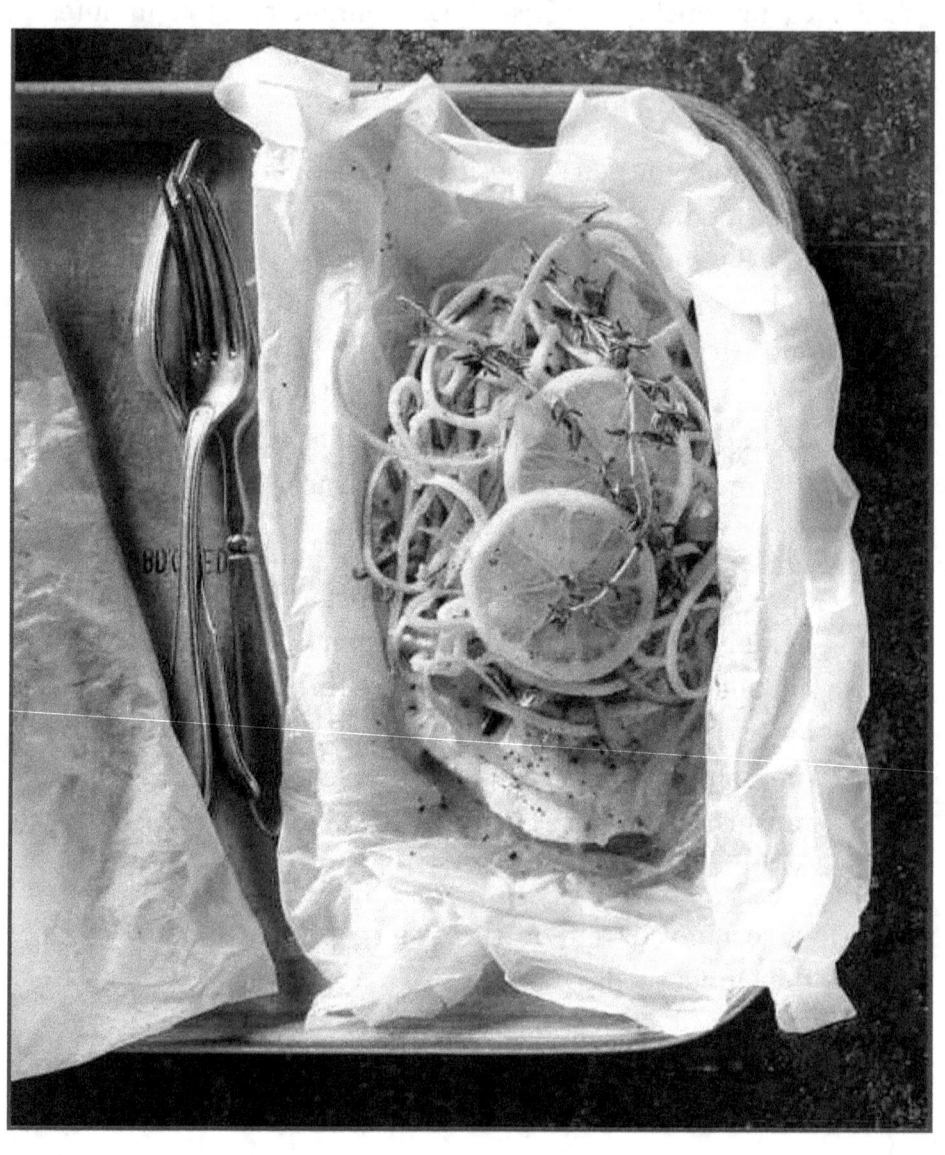

SOLE EN PAPILLOTE WITH JULIENNE VEGETABLES

PREP: 30 minutes BAKE: 12 minutes MAKES: 4 servings PHOTO

YOU CAN CERTAINLY JULIENNE VEGETABLES WITH A GOOD SHARP CHEF'S KNIFE, BUT IT IS VERY TIME-CONSUMING. A JULIENNE PEELER (SEE "EQUIPMENT") MAKES QUICK WORK OF CREATING LONG, THIN, CONSISENTLY SHAPED STRIPS OF VEGETABLES.

4 6-ounce fresh or frozen sole, flounder, or other firm white fish fillets

1 zucchini, julienne cut

1 large carrot, julienne cut

½ of a red onion, julienne cut

2 roma tomatoes, seeded and finely chopped

2 cloves garlic, minced

1 tablespoon olive oil

½ teaspoon black pepper

1 lemon, cut into 8 thin slices, seeds removed

8 sprigs fresh thyme

4 teaspoons olive oil

¼ cup dry white wine

1. Thaw fish, if frozen. Preheat oven to 375°F. In a large bowl combine zucchini, carrot, onion, tomatoes, and garlic. Add 1 tablespoon olive oil and ¼ teaspoon of the pepper; toss well to combine. Set vegetables aside.

2. Cut four 14-inch squares of parchment paper. Rinse fish; pat dry with paper towels. Place a fillet in the center of each square. Sprinkle with the remaining ¼ teaspoon pepper. Arrange vegetables, lemon slices, and thyme sprigs on top

of fillets, dividing evenly. Drizzle each stack with 1 teaspoon olive oil and 1 tablespoon white wine.

3. Working with one packet at a time, bring up two opposite sides of the parchment paper and fold together several times over fish. Fold ends of parchment to seal.

4. Arrange packets on a large baking sheet. Bake about 12 minutes or until fish begins to flake when tested with a fork (carefully open packet to check doneness).

5. To serve, place each packet on a dinner plate; carefully open packets.

ARUGULA PESTO FISH TACOS WITH SMOKY LIME CREAM

PREP: 30 minutes GRILL: 4 to 6 minutes per ½-inch thickness MAKES: 6 servings

YOU CAN SUBSTITUTE COD FOR THE SOLE—JUST NOT TILAPIA. TILAPIA IS UNFORTUNATELY ONE OF THE WORST CHOICES FOR FISH. IT IS ALMOST UNIVERSALLY FARM-RAISED AND FREQUENTLY UNDER HORRIBLE CONDITIONS—SO WHILE TILAPIA IS NEARLY UBIQUITOUS, IT SHOULD BE AVOIDED.

   4 4- to 5-ounce fresh or frozen sole fillets, about ½ inch thick
   1 recipe Arugula Pesto (see recipe)
   ½ cup Cashew Cream (see recipe)
   1 teaspoon Smoky Seasoning (see recipe)
   ½ teaspoon finely shredded lime peel
   12 butterhead lettuce leaves
   1 ripe avocado, halved, seeded, peeled, and cut into thin slices
   1 cup chopped tomato
   ¼ cup snipped fresh cilantro
   1 lime, cut into wedges

1. Thaw fish, if frozen. Rinse fish; pat dry with paper towels. Set fish aside.

2. Rub some of the Arugula Pesto on both sides of the fish.

3. For a charcoal or gas grill, place fish on a greased rack directly over medium heat. Cover and grill for 4 to 6 minutes or until fish begins to flake when tested with a fork, turning once halfway through grilling.

4. Meanwhile, for Smoky Lime Cream, in a small bowl stir together the Cashew Cream, Smoky Seasoning, and lime peel.

5. Using a fork, break fish into pieces. Fill butterhead leaves with fish, avocado slices, and tomato; sprinkle with cilantro. Drizzle tacos with Smoky Lime Cream. Serve with lime wedges to squeeze over tacos.

ALMOND-CRUSTED SOLE

PREP: 15 minutes COOK: 3 minutes MAKES: 2 servings

JUST A LITTLE BIT OF ALMOND FLOUR CREATES A NICE CRUST ON THIS EXTREMELY QUICK-COOKING PAN-FRIED FISH SERVED WITH CREAMY DILLED MAYONNAISE AND A SQUEEZE OF FRESH LEMON.

12 ounces fresh or frozen sole fillets
1 tablespoon Lemon-Herb Seasoning (see recipe)
¼ to ½ teaspoon black pepper
⅓ cup almond flour
2 to 3 tablespoons olive oil
¼ cup Paleo Mayo (see recipe)
1 teaspoon snipped fresh dill
Lemon wedges

1. Thaw fish, if frozen. Rinse fish; pat dry with paper towels. In a small bowl stir together the Lemon-Herb Seasoning and pepper. Coat both sides of fillets with seasoning mixture, pressing lightly to adhere. Spread almond flour on a large plate. Dredge one side of each fillet in the almond flour, pressing lightly to adhere.

2. In a large skillet heat enough oil to coat pan over medium-high heat. Add fish, coated sides down. Cook for 2 minutes. Carefully turn fish over; cook about 1 minute more or until the fish begins to flake when tested with a fork.

3. For sauce, in a small bowl stir together the Paleo Mayo and dill. Serve fish with sauce and lemon wedges.

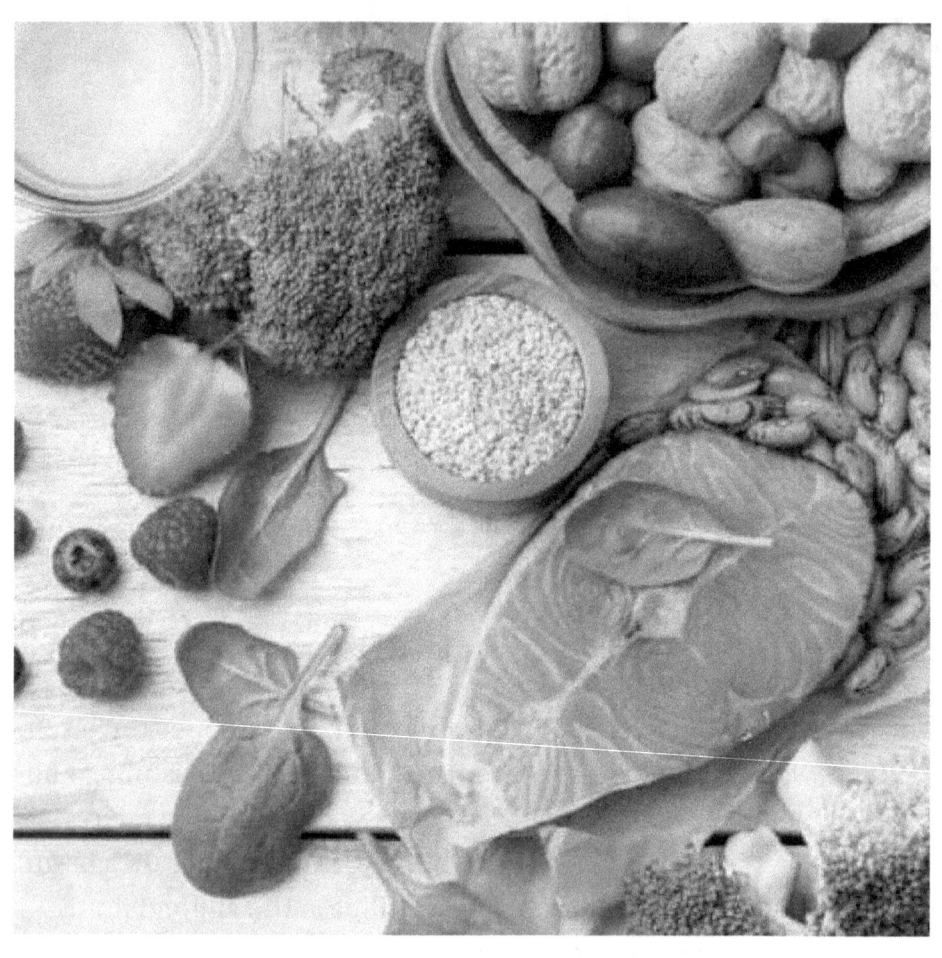

GRILLED COD AND ZUCCHINI PACKETS WITH SPICY MANGO-BASIL SAUCE

PREP: 20 minutes GRILL: 6 minutes MAKES: 4 servings

1 to 1½ pounds fresh or frozen cod, ½ to 1 inch thick
4 24-inch-long pieces 12-inch-wide foil
1 medium zucchini, cut into julienne strips
Lemon-Herb Seasoning (see recipe)
¼ cup Chipotle Paleo Mayo (see recipe)
1 to 2 tablespoons pureed ripe mango*
1 tablespoon fresh lime or lemon juice or rice wine vinegar
2 tablespoons snipped fresh basil

1. Thaw fish, if frozen. Rinse fish; pat dry with paper towels. Cut fish into four serving-size pieces.

2. Fold each piece of foil in half to create a double-thickness 12-inch square. Place one portion of fish in the middle of a foil square. Top with one-fourth of the zucchini. Sprinkle with Lemon-Herb Seasoning. Bring up two opposite sides of foil and fold several times over zucchini and fish. Fold ends of foil. Repeat to make three more packets. For sauce, in a small bowl stir together Chipotle Paleo Mayo, mango, lime juice, and basil; set aside.

3. For a charcoal grill or gas grill, place packets on the oiled grill rack directly over medium heat. Cover and grill for 6 to 9 minutes or until fish begins to flake when tested with a fork and zucchini is crisp-tender (carefully open packet to test doneness). Do not turn packets while grilling. Top each serving with sauce.

*Tip: For mango puree, in a blender combine ¼ cup chopped mango and 1 tablespoon water. Cover and blend until smooth. Add any leftover pureed mango to a smoothie.

RIESLING-POACHED COD WITH PESTO-STUFFED TOMATOES

PREP: 30 minutes COOK: 10 minutes MAKES: 4 servings

1 to 1½ pounds fresh or frozen cod fillets, about 1 inch thick

4 roma tomatoes

3 tablespoons Basil Pesto (see recipe)

¼ teaspoon cracked black pepper

1 cup dry Riesling or Sauvignon Blanc

1 sprig fresh thyme or ½ teaspoon dried thyme, crushed

1 bay leaf

½ cup water

2 tablespoons chopped scallion

Lemon wedges

1. Thaw fish, if frozen. Cut tomatoes in half horizontally. Scoop out the seeds and some of the flesh. (If necessary for tomato to sit flat, cut a very thin slice off the end, being careful not to make a hole in the bottom of the tomato.) Spoon some pesto into each tomato half; sprinkle with cracked pepper; set aside.

2. Rinse fish; pat dry with paper towels. Cut fish into four pieces. Place a steamer basket in a large skillet with a tight-fitting lid. Add about ½ inch water to skillet. Bring to boiling; reduce heat to medium. Add the tomatoes, cut sides up, to the basket. Cover and steam for 2 to 3 minutes or until warmed through.

3. Remove tomatoes to a plate; cover to keep warm. Remove steamer basket from skillet; discard water. Add wine, thyme, bay leaf, and the ½ cup water to skillet. Bring to boiling; reduce heat to medium-low. Add fish and scallion.

Simmer, covered, for 8 to 10 minutes or until fish begins to flake when tested with a fork.

4. Drizzle fish with some of the poaching liquid. Serve fish with pesto-stuffed tomatoes and lemon wedges.

BROILED PISTACHIO-CILANTRO-CRUSTED COD OVER SMASHED SWEET POTATOES

PREP: 20 minutes COOK: 10 minutes BROIL: 4 to 6 minutes per ½-inch thickness MAKES: 4 servings

- 1 to 1½ pounds fresh or frozen cod
- Olive oil or refined coconut oil
- 2 tablespoons ground pistachios, pecans, or almonds
- 1 egg white
- ½ teaspoon finely shredded lemon peel
- 1½ pounds sweet potatoes, peeled and cut into chunks
- 2 cloves garlic
- 1 tablespoon coconut oil
- 1 tablespoon grated fresh ginger
- ½ teaspoon ground cumin
- ¼ cup coconut milk (such as Nature's Way)
- 4 teaspoons Cilantro Pesto or Basil Pesto (see recipes)

1. Thaw fish, if frozen. Preheat broiler. Oil rack of a broiler pan. In a small bowl combine ground nuts, egg white, and lemon peel; set aside.

2. For the smashed sweet potatoes, in a medium saucepan cook sweet potatoes and garlic in enough boiling water to cover for 10 to 15 minutes or until tender. Drain; return sweet potatoes and garlic to the saucepan. Using a potato masher, mash sweet potatoes. Stir in 1 tablespoon coconut oil, ginger, and cumin. Mash in coconut milk until light and fluffy.

3. Rinse fish; pat dry with paper towels. Cut fish into four pieces and place on the prepared unheated rack of a

broiler pan. Tuck under any thin edges. Spread each piece with Cilantro Pesto. Spoon nut mixture on pesto and spread gently. Broil fish 4 inches from the heat for 4 to 6 minutes per ½-inch thickness or until fish begins to flake when tested with a fork, covering with foil during broiling if coating starts to burn. Serve fish with sweet potatoes.

ROSEMARY-AND-TANGERINE COD WITH ROASTED BROCCOLI

PREP: 15 minutes MARINATE: up to 30 minutes BAKE: 12 minutes MAKES: 4 servings

1 to 1½ pounds fresh or frozen cod
1 teaspoon finely shredded tangerine peel
½ cup fresh tangerine or orange juice
4 tablespoons olive oil
2 teaspoons snipped fresh rosemary
¼ to ½ teaspoon cracked black pepper
1 teaspoon finely shredded tangerine peel
3 cups broccoli florets
¼ teaspoon crushed red pepper
Tangerine slices, seeds removed

1. Preheat oven to 450°F. Thaw fish, if frozen. Rinse fish; pat dry with paper towels. Cut fish into four serving-size pieces. Measure thickness of fish. In a shallow dish combine tangerine peel, tangerine juice, 2 tablespoons of the olive oil, rosemary, and black pepper; add fish. Cover and marinate in the refrigerator for up to 30 minutes.

2. In a large bowl toss broccoli with the remaining 2 tablespoons olive oil and the crushed red pepper. Place in a 2-quart baking dish.

3. Brush a shallow baking pan lightly with additional olive oil. Drain fish, reserving marinade. Place fish in the pan, tucking under any thin edges. Place fish and broccoli in the oven. Bake broccoli for 12 to 15 minutes or until crisp-tender, stirring once halfway through cooking. Bake fish for 4 to 6 minutes per ½-inch thickness of fish or until fish begins to flake when tested with a fork.

4. In a small saucepan bring reserved marinade to boiling; cook for 2 minutes. Drizzle the marinade over the cooked fish. Serve fish with broccoli and tangerine slices.

CURRIED COD LETTUCE WRAPS WITH PICKLED RADISHES

PREP: 20 minutes STAND: 20 minutes COOK: 6 minutes MAKES: 4 servings PHOTO

- 1 pound fresh or frozen cod fillets
- 6 radishes, coarsely shredded
- 6 to 7 tablespoons cider vinegar
- ½ teaspoon crushed red pepper
- 2 tablespoons unrefined coconut oil
- ¼ cup almond butter
- 1 clove garlic, minced
- 2 teaspoons finely grated ginger
- 2 tablespoons olive oil
- 1½ to 2 teaspoons no-salt-added curry powder
- 4 to 8 butterhead lettuce leaves or leaf lettuce leaves
- 1 red sweet pepper, cut into julienne strips
- 2 tablespoons snipped fresh cilantro

1. Thaw fish, if frozen. In a medium bowl combine radishes, 4 tablespoons of the vinegar, and ¼ teaspoon of the crushed red pepper; let stand for 20 minutes, stirring occasionally.

2. For almond butter sauce, in a small saucepan melt the coconut oil over low heat. Stir in almond butter until smooth. Stir in garlic, ginger, and remaining ¼ teaspoon crushed red pepper. Remove from heat. Add the remaining 2 to 3 tablespoons cider vinegar, stirring until smooth; set aside. (Sauce will thicken slightly when vinegar is added.)

3. Rinse fish; pat dry with paper towels. In a large skillet heat the olive oil and curry powder over medium heat. Add fish; cook for 3 to 6 minutes or until fish begins to flake

when tested with a fork, turning once halfway through cooking time. Using two forks, coarsely flake fish.

4. Drain radishes; discard marinade. Spoon some of the fish, sweet pepper strips, radish mixture, and almond butter sauce into each lettuce leaf. Sprinkle with cilantro. Wrap leaf around filling. If desired, secure wraps with wooden toothpicks.

ROASTED HADDOCK WITH LEMON AND FENNEL

PREP: 25 minutes ROAST: 50 minutes MAKES: 4 servings

HADDOCK, POLLOCK, AND COD ALL HAVE MILDLY FLAVORED FIRM WHITE FLESH. THEY ARE INTERCHANGEABLE IN MOST RECIPES, INCLUDING THIS SIMPLE DISH OF BAKED FISH AND VEGETABLES WITH HERBS AND WINE.

4 6-ounce fresh or frozen haddock, pollock, or cod fillets, about ½ inch thick

1 large bulb fennel, cored and sliced, fronds reserved and chopped

4 medium carrots, cut in half vertically and sliced into 2- to 3-inch-long pieces

1 red onion, halved and sliced

2 cloves garlic, minced

1 lemon, thinly sliced

3 tablespoons olive oil

½ teaspoon black pepper

¾ cup dry white wine

2 tablespoons finely snipped fresh parsley

2 tablespoons snipped fresh fennel fronds

2 teaspoons finely shredded lemon peel

1. Thaw fish, if frozen. Preheat oven to 400°F. In a 3-quart rectangular baking dish combine fennel, carrots, onion, garlic, and lemon slices. Drizzle with 2 tablespoons of the olive oil and sprinkle with ¼ teaspoon of the pepper; toss to coat. Pour wine into dish. Cover dish with foil.

2. Roast for 20 minutes. Uncover; stir vegetable mixture. Roast 15 to 20 minutes more or until vegetables are crisp-tender. Stir vegetable mixture. Sprinkle fish with the remaining ¼ teaspoon pepper; place fish on top of vegetable mixture. Drizzle with the remaining 1

tablespoon olive oil. Roast about 8 to 10 minutes or until fish begins to flake when tested with a fork.

3. In a small bowl combine parsley, fennel fronds, and lemon peel. To serve, divide fish and vegetable mixture among serving plates. Spoon pan juices over fish and vegetables. Sprinkle with parsley mixture.

PECAN-CRUSTED SNAPPER WITH REMOULADE AND CAJUN-STYLE OKRA AND TOMATOES

PREP: 1 hour COOK: 10 minutes BAKE: 8 minutes MAKES: 4 servings

THIS COMPANY-WORTHY FISH DISH TAKES A BIT OF TIME TO MAKE, BUT THE RICH FLAVORS MAKE IT WELL WORTH IT. THE REMOULADE—A MAYONNAISE-BASED SAUCE SPIKED WITH MUSTARD, LEMON, AND CAJUN SEASONING AND CONFETTIED WITH CHOPPED RED SWEET PEPPER, SCALLIONS, AND PARSLEY—CAN BE MADE A DAY AHEAD AND CHILLED.

- 4 tablespoons olive oil
- ½ cup finely chopped pecans
- 2 tablespoons chopped fresh parsley
- 1 tablespoon chopped fresh thyme
- 2 8-ounce red snapper fillets, ½ inch thick
- 4 teaspoons Cajun Seasoning (see recipe)
- ½ cup diced onion
- ½ cup diced green sweet pepper
- ½ cup diced celery
- 1 tablespoon minced garlic
- 1 pound fresh okra pods, cut into 1-inch-thick slices (or fresh asparagus, cut into 1-inch lengths)
- 8 ounces grape or cherry tomatoes, halved
- 2 teaspoons chopped fresh thyme
- Black pepper
- Rémoulade (see recipe, right)

1. In a medium skillet heat 1 tablespoon of the olive oil over medium heat. Add the pecans and toast about 5 minutes or until golden and fragrant, stirring frequently. Transfer

pecans to a small bowl and let cool. Add parsley and thyme and set aside.

2. Preheat oven to 400°F. Line a baking sheet with parchment paper or foil. Arrange the snapper fillets on the baking sheet, skin sides down, and sprinkle each with 1 teaspoon of the Cajun Seasoning. Using a pastry brush, dab 2 tablespoons of olive oil onto fillets. Divide the pecan mixture evenly among the fillets, pressing the nuts gently onto the surface of the fish so they adhere. Cover all the exposed areas of the fish fillet with nuts if possible. Bake fish for 8 to 10 minutes or until it flakes easily with the tip of a knife.

3. In a large skillet heat the remaining 1 tablespoon olive oil over medium-high heat. Add onion, sweet pepper, celery, and garlic. Cook and stir for 5 minutes or until vegetables are crisp-tender. Add the sliced okra (or asparagus if using) and the tomatoes; cook for 5 to 7 minutes or until okra is crisp-tender and tomatoes begin to split. Remove from heat and season with thyme and black pepper to taste. Serve vegetables with snapper and Rémoulade.

Remoulade: In a food processor pulse ½ cup chopped red sweet pepper, ¼ cup chopped scallions, and 2 tablespoons chopped fresh parsley until fine. Add ¼ cup Paleo Mayo (see recipe), ¼ cup Dijon-Style Mustard (see recipe), 1½ teaspoons lemon juice, and ¼ teaspoon Cajun Seasoning (see recipe). Pulse until combined. Transfer to a serving bowl and refrigerate until ready to serve. (Remoulade may be made 1 day ahead and chilled.)

TARRAGON TUNA PATTIES WITH AVOCADO-LEMON AÏOLI

PREP: 25 minutes COOK: 6 minutes MAKES: 4 servings PHOTO

ALONG WITH SALMON, TUNA IS ONE OF THE RARE KINDS OF FISH THAT CAN BE FINELY CHOPPED AND FORMED INTO BURGERS. BE CAREFUL NOT TO OVERPROCESS THE TUNA IN THE FOOD PROCESSOR—OVERPROCESSING TOUGHENS IT.

1 pound fresh or frozen skinless tuna fillets

1 egg white, lightly beaten

¾ cup ground golden flaxseed meal

1 tablespoon fresh snipped tarragon or dill

2 tablespoons snipped fresh chives

1 teaspoon finely shredded lemon peel

2 tablespoons flaxseed oil, avocado oil, or olive oil

1 medium avocado, seeded

3 tablespoons Paleo Mayo (see recipe)

1 teaspoon finely shredded lemon peel

2 teaspoons fresh lemon juice

1 clove garlic, minced

4 ounces baby spinach (about 4 cups tightly packed)

⅓ cup Roasted Garlic Vinaigrette (see recipe)

1 Granny Smith apple, cored and cut into matchstick-size pieces

¼ cup chopped toasted walnuts (see tip)

1. Thaw fish, if frozen. Rinse fish; pat dry with paper towels. Cut fish into 1½-inch pieces. Place fish in a food processor; process with on/off pulses until finely chopped. (Be careful not to overprocess or you'll toughen the patty.) Set fish aside.

2. In a medium bowl combine egg white, ¼ cup of the flaxseed meal, tarragon, chives, and lemon peel. Add fish; stir gently to combine. Shape fish mixture into four ½-inch-thick patties.

3. Place remaining ½ cup flaxseed meal in a shallow dish. Dip patties into flaxseed mixture, turning to coat evenly.

4. In an extra-large skillet heat oil over medium heat. Cook tuna patties in hot oil for 6 to 8 minutes or until an instant-read thermometer inserted horizontally into patties registers 160°F, turning once halfway through cooking time.

5. Meanwhile, for the aïoli, in a medium bowl use a fork to mash avocado. Add Paleo Mayo, lemon peel, lemon juice, and garlic. Mash until well mixed and almost smooth.

6. Place the spinach in a medium bowl. Drizzle spinach with Roasted Garlic Vinaigrette; toss to coat. For each serving, place a tuna patty and one-fourth of the spinach on a serving plate. Top tuna with some of the aïoli. Top spinach with apple and walnuts. Serve immediately.

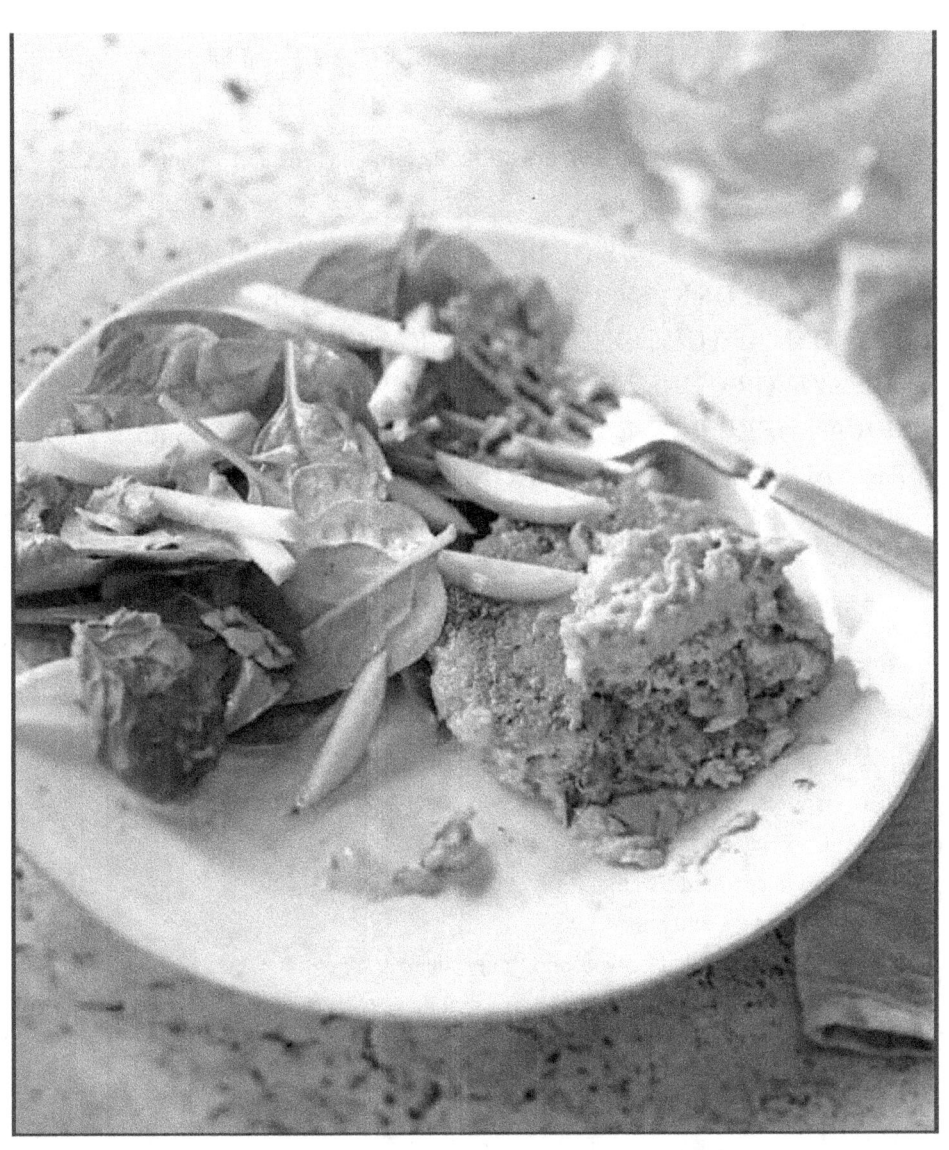

STRIPED BASS TAGINE

PREP: 50 minutes CHILL: 1 to 2 hours COOK: 22 minutes BAKE: 25 minutes MAKES: 4 servings

A TAGINE IS THE NAME OF BOTH A TYPE OF NORTH AFRICAN DISH (A KIND OF STEW) AND THE CONE-SHAPE POT IT'S COOKED IN. IF YOU DON'T HAVE ONE, A COVERED OVEN-GOING SKILLET WORKS JUST FINE. CHERMOULA IS A THICK NORTH AFRICAN HERB PASTE THAT IS MOST OFTEN USED AS A MARINADE FOR FISH. SERVE THIS COLORFUL FISH DISH WITH A SWEET POTATO OR CAULIFLOWER MASH.

- 4 6-ounce fresh or frozen striped bass or halibut fillets, skin on
- 1 bunch cilantro, chopped
- 1 teaspoon finely shredded lemon peel (set aside)
- ¼ cup fresh lemon juice
- 4 tablespoons olive oil
- 5 cloves garlic, minced
- 4 teaspoons ground cumin
- 2 teaspoons sweet paprika
- 1 teaspoon ground coriander
- ¼ teaspoon ground anise
- 1 large onion, peeled, halved, and thinly sliced
- 1 15-ounce can no-salt-added fire-roasted diced tomatoes, undrained
- ½ cup Chicken Bone Broth (see recipe) or no-salt-added chicken broth
- 1 large yellow sweet pepper, seeded and cut into ½-inch- strips
- 1 large orange sweet pepper, seeded and cut into ½-inch strips

1. Thaw fish, if frozen. Rinse fish; pat dry with paper towels. Place fish fillets in a shallow, nonmetal baking dish. Set fish aside.

2. For chermoula, in a blender or small food processor combine cilantro, lemon juice, 2 tablespoons of the olive

oil, 4 cloves minced garlic, the cumin, paprika, coriander, and anise. Cover and process until smooth.

3. Spoon half of the chermoula over the fish, turning fish to coat both sides. Cover and refrigerate for 1 to 2 hours. Cover remaining chermoula; let stand at room temperature until needed.

4. Preheat oven to 325°F. In a large oven-going skillet heat the remaining 2 tablespoons oil over medium-high heat. Add onion; cook and stir for 4 to 5 minutes or until tender. Stir in the remaining 1 clove minced garlic; cook and stir for 1 minute. Add reserved chermoula, tomatoes, Chicken Bone Broth, sweet pepper strips, and lemon peel. Bring to boiling; reduce heat. Simmer, uncovered, for 15 minutes. If desired, transfer mixture to tagine; top with fish and any remaining chermoula from the dish. Cover; bake for 25 minutes. Serve immediately.

HALIBUT IN GARLIC-SHRIMP SAUCE WITH SOFFRITO COLLARD GREENS

PREP: 30 minutes COOK: 19 minutes MAKES: 4 servings

THERE ARE SEVERAL DIFFERENT SOURCES AND TYPES OF HALIBUT, AND THEY CAN BE OF VASTLY DIFFERENT QUALITY—AND FISHED UNDER VERY DIFFERENT CONDITIONS. THE SUSTAINABILITY OF THE FISH, THE ENVIRONMENT IN WHICH IT LIVES, AND THE CONDITIONS UNDER WHICH IT IS RAISED/FISHED ARE ALL FACTORS IN DETERMINING WHICH FISH ARE GOOD CHOICES FOR CONSUMPTION. VISIT THE MONTEREY BAY AQUARIUM WEBSITE (WWW.SEAFOODWATCH.ORG) FOR THE LATEST INFORMATION ON WHICH FISH TO EAT AND WHICH ONES TO AVOID.

- 4 6-ounce fresh or frozen halibut fillets, about 1 inch thick
- Black pepper
- 6 tablespoons extra virgin olive oil
- ½ cup finely chopped onion
- ¼ cup diced red sweet pepper
- 2 cloves garlic, minced
- ¾ teaspoon smoked Spanish paprika
- ½ teaspoon chopped fresh oregano
- 4 cups collard greens, stemmed, sliced into ¼-inch-thick ribbons (about 12 ounces)
- ⅓ cup water
- 8 ounces medium shrimp, peeled, deveined, and coarsely chopped
- 4 cloves garlic, thinly sliced
- ¼ to ½ teaspoon crushed red pepper
- ⅓ cup dry sherry
- 2 tablespoons lemon juice
- ¼ cup chopped fresh parsley

1. Thaw fish, if frozen. Rinse fish; pat dry with paper towels. Sprinkle fish with pepper. In a large skillet heat 2 tablespoons of the olive oil over medium heat. Add the fillets; cook for 10 minutes or until golden brown and fish flakes when tested with a fork, turning once halfway through cooking. Transfer the fish to a platter and tent with foil to keep warm.

2. Meanwhile, in another large skillet heat 1 tablespoon of the olive oil over medium heat. Add onion, sweet pepper, 2 cloves minced garlic, paprika, and oregano; cook and stir for 3 to 5 minutes or until tender. Stir in collard greens and the water. Cover and cook for 3 to 4 minutes or until liquid has evaporated and greens are just tender, stirring occasionally. Cover and keep warm until ready to serve.

3. For shrimp sauce, add remaining 3 tablespoons olive oil to the skillet used for cooking the fish. Add the shrimp, 4 cloves sliced garlic, and crushed red pepper. Cook and stir for 2 to 3 minutes or until garlic just begins to turn golden. Add the shrimp; cook for 2 to 3 minutes until shrimp is firm and pink. Stir in the sherry and lemon juice. Cook 1 to 2 minutes or until reduced slightly. Stir in the parsley.

4. Divide shrimp sauce among halibut fillets. Serve with greens.

SEAFOOD BOUILLABAISSE

START TO FINISH: 1¾ hours MAKES: 4 servings

LIKE ITALIAN CIOPPINO, THIS FRENCH SEAFOOD STEW OF FISH AND SHELLFISH SEEMS TO REPRESENT A SAMPLING OF THE DAY'S CATCH THROWN INTO A POT WITH GARLIC, ONIONS, TOMATOES, AND WINE. THE DISTINGUISHING FLAVOR OF BOUILLABAISSE, HOWEVER, IS THE FLAVOR COMBINATION OF SAFFRON, FENNEL, AND ORANGE ZEST.

1 pound fresh or frozen skinless halibut fillet, cut into 1-inch pieces
4 tablespoons olive oil
2 cups chopped onions
4 cloves garlic, smashed
1 head fennel, cored and chopped
6 roma tomatoes, chopped
¾ cup Chicken Bone Broth (see recipe) or no-salt-added chicken broth
¼ cup dry white wine
1 cup finely chopped onion
1 head fennel, cored and finely chopped
6 cloves garlic, minced
1 orange
3 roma tomatoes, finely chopped
4 saffron threads
1 tablespoon snipped fresh oregano
1 pound littleneck clams, scrubbed and rinsed
1 pound mussels, beards removed, scrubbed, and rinsed (see tip)
Snipped fresh oregano (optional)

1. Thaw halibut, if frozen. Rinse fish; pat dry with paper towels. Set fish aside.

2. In a 6- to 8-quart Dutch oven, heat 2 tablespoons of the olive oil over medium heat. Add 2 cups chopped onions, 1 head

chopped fennel, and 4 cloves smashed garlic to the pot. Cook for 7 to 9 minutes or until onion is tender, stirring occasionally. Add 6 chopped tomatoes and 1 head chopped fennel; cook for 4 minutes more. Add Chicken Bone Broth and white wine to pot; simmer for 5 minutes; cool slightly. Transfer vegetable mixture to a blender or food processor. Cover and blend or process until smooth; set aside.

3. In the same Dutch oven heat the remaining 1 tablespoon olive oil over medium heat. Add 1 cup finely chopped onion, 1 head finely chopped fennel, and 6 cloves minced garlic. Cook over medium heat 5 to 7 minutes or until nearly tender, stirring frequently.

4. Use a vegetable peeler to remove the zest from the orange in wide strips; set aside. Add the pureed vegetable mixture, 3 chopped tomatoes, saffron, oregano, and orange zest strips to the Dutch oven. Bring to boiling; reduce heat to maintain simmering. Add clams, mussels, and fish; stir gently to coat fish with sauce. Adjust heat as needned to maintain a simmer. Cover and simmer gently for 3 to 5 minutes until mussels and clams have opened and fish begins to flake when tested with a fork. Ladle into shallow bowls to serve. If desired, sprinkle with additional oregano.

CLASSIC SHRIMP CEVICHE

PREP: 20 minutes COOK: 2 minutes CHILL: 1 hour STAND: 30 minutes MAKES: 3 to 4 servings

THIS LATIN AMERICAN DISH IS AN EXPLOSION OF TASTES AND TEXTURES. CRUNCHY CUCUMBER AND CELERY, CREAMY AVOCADO, HOT AND SPICY JALAPEÑOS, AND DELICATE, SWEET SHRIMP INTERMINGLE IN LIME JUICE AND OLIVE OIL. IN TRADITIONAL CEVICHE, THE ACID IN THE LIME JUICE "COOKS" THE SHRIMP—BUT A QUICK DIP IN BOILING WATER LEAVES NOTHING TO CHANCE, SAFETYWISE—AND DOESN'T HURT THE FLAVOR OR TEXTURE OF THE SHRIMP.

- 1 pound fresh or frozen medium shrimp, peeled and deveined, tails removed
- ½ of a cucumber, peeled, seeded, and chopped
- 1 cup chopped celery
- ½ of a small red onion, chopped
- 1 to 2 jalapeños, seeded and minced (see tip)
- ½ cup fresh lime juice
- 2 roma tomatoes, diced
- 1 avocado, halved, seeded, peeled, and diced
- ¼ cup snipped fresh cilantro
- 3 tablespoons olive oil
- ½ teaspoon black pepper

1. Thaw shrimp, if frozen. Peel and devein shrimp; remove tails. Rinse shrimp; pat dry with paper towels.

2. Fill a large saucepan half full with water. Bring to boiling. Add shrimp to boiling water. Cook, uncovered, for 1 to 2 minutes or just until shrimp turn opaque; drain. Run shrimp under cool water and drain again. Dice shrimp.

3. In a extra-large nonreactive bowl combine shrimp, cucumber, celery, onion, jalapeños, and lime juice. Cover and refrigerate for 1 hour, stirring once or twice.

4. Stir in tomatoes, avocado, cilantro, olive oil, and black pepper. Cover and let stand at room temperature for 30 minutes. Stir gently before serving.

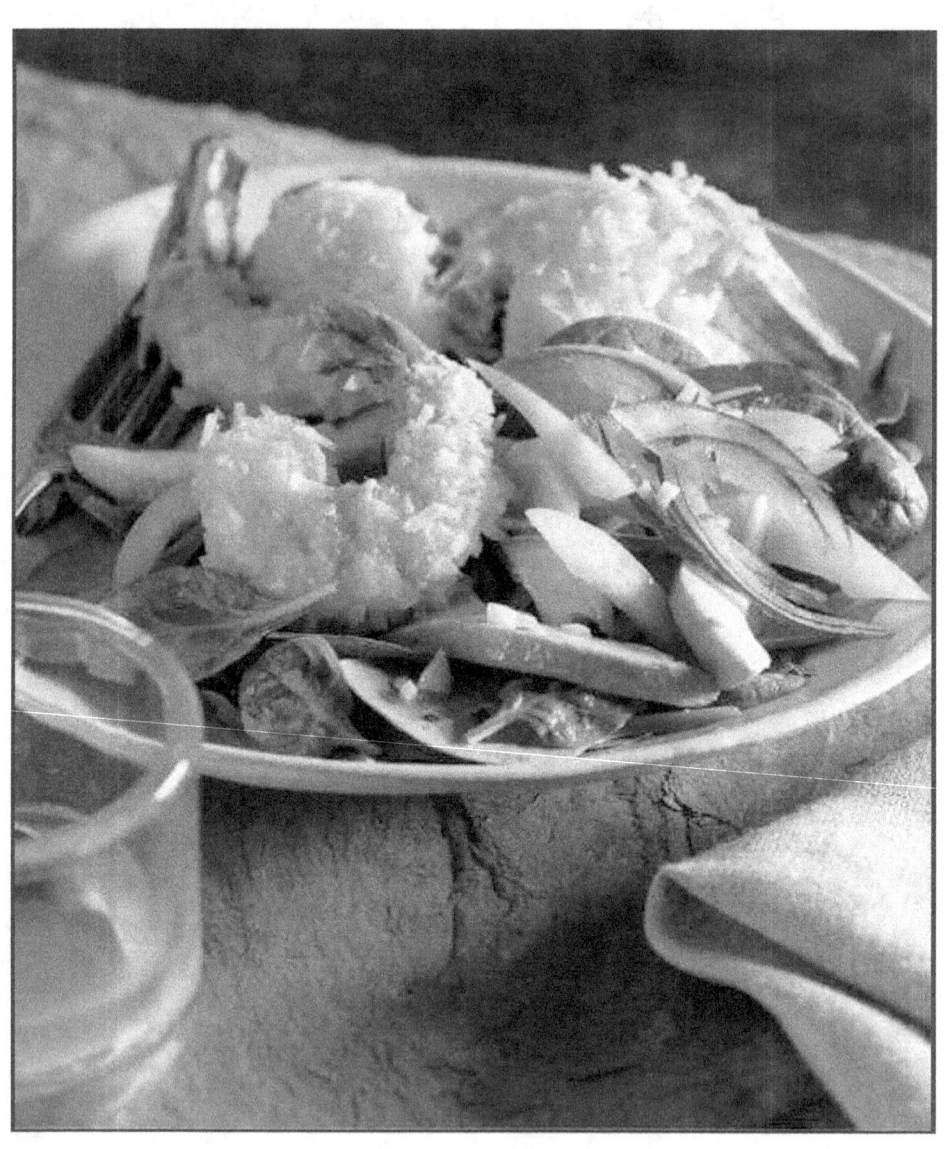

COCONUT-CRUSTED SHRIMP AND SPINACH SALAD

PREP: 25 minutes BAKE: 8 minutes MAKES: 4 servings PHOTO

COMMERCIALLY PRODUCED CANS OF SPRAY OLIVE OIL CAN CONTAIN GRAIN ALCOHOL, LECITHIN, AND PROPELLANT—NOT A TERRIFIC MIX WHEN YOU ARE TRYING TO EAT PURE, REAL FOODS AND AVOID GRAINS, UNHEALTHY FATS, LEGUMES, AND DAIRY. AN OIL MISTER USES ONLY AIR TO PROPEL THE OIL INTO A FINE SPRAY—PERFECT FOR LIGHTLY COATING COCONUT-CRUSTED SHRIMP BEFORE BAKING.

- 1½ pounds fresh or frozen extra-large shrimp in shells
- Misto spray bottle filled with extra virgin olive oil
- 2 eggs
- ¾ cup unsweetened flaked or shredded coconut
- ¾ cup almond meal
- ½ cup avocado oil or olive oil
- 3 tablespoons fresh lemon juice
- 2 tablespoons fresh lime juice
- 2 small cloves garlic, minced
- ⅛ to ¼ teaspoon crushed red pepper
- 8 cups fresh baby spinach
- 1 medium avocado, halved, seeded, peeled, and thinly sliced
- 1 small orange or yellow sweet pepper, cut into thin bite-size strips
- ½ cup slivered red onion

1. Thaw shrimp, if frozen. Peel and devein shrimp, leaving tails intact. Rinse shrimp; pat dry with paper towels. Preheat oven to 450°F. Line a large baking sheet with foil; lightly coat foil with oil sprayed from the Misto bottle; set aside.

2. In a shallow dish beat eggs with a fork. In another shallow dish combine coconut and almond meal. Dip shrimp into eggs, turning to coat. Dip in coconut mixture, pressing to coat (leave tails uncoated). Arrange shrimp in a single layer on the prepared baking sheet. Coat the tops of the shrimp with oil sprayed from the Misto bottle.

3. Bake for 8 to 10 minutes or until shrimp are opaque and coating is lightly browned.

4. Meanwhile, for dressing, in a small screw-top jar combine avocado oil, lemon juice, lime juice, garlic, and crushed red pepper. Cover and shake well.

5. For salads, divide spinach among four serving plates. Top with avocado, sweet pepper, red onion, and the shrimp. Drizzle with dressing and serve immediately.

TROPICAL SHRIMP AND SCALLOP CEVICHE

PREP: 20 minutes MARINATE: 30 to 60 minutes MAKES: 4 to 6 servings

COOL AND LIGHT CEVICHE MAKES A GREAT MEAL FOR A HOT SUMMER NIGHT. WITH MELON, MANGO, SERRANO CHILES, FENNEL, AND MANGO-LIME SALAD DRESSING (SEE RECIPE), THIS IS A SWEET-HOT TAKE ON THE ORIGINAL.

1 pound fresh or frozen sea scallops
1 pound fresh or frozen large shrimp
2 cups cubed honeydew melon
2 medium mangoes, pitted, peeled, and chopped (about 2 cups)
1 head fennel, trimmed, quartered, cored, and thinly sliced
1 medium red sweet pepper, chopped (about ¾ cup)
1 to 2 serrano chiles, seeded if desired and thinly sliced (see tip)
½ cup lightly packed fresh cilantro, chopped
1 recipe Mango-Lime Salad Dressing (see recipe)

1. Thaw scallops and shrimp, if frozen. Split scallops in half horizontally. Peel, devein, and split shrimp in half horizontally. Rinse scallops and shrimp; pat dry with paper towels. Fill a large saucepan three-fourths full with water. Bring to boiling. Add shrimp and scallops; cook for 3 to 4 minutes or until shrimp and scallops are opaque; drain and rinse with cold water to cool quickly. Drain well and set aside.

2. In an extra-large bowl combine melon, mangoes, fennel, sweet pepper, serrano chiles, and cilantro. Add Mango-Lime Salad Dressing; toss gently to coat. Gently stir in

JAMAICAN JERK SHRIMP WITH AVOCADO OIL

START TO FINISH: 20 minutes MAKES: 4 servings

WITH A TOTAL TO-THE-TABLE TIME OF 20 MINUTES, THIS DISH OFFERS ONE MORE COMPELLING REASON TO EAT A HEALTHY MEAL AT HOME, EVEN ON THE BUSIEST NIGHTS.

- 1 pound fresh or frozen medium shrimp
- 1 cup chopped, peeled mango (1 medium)
- ⅓ cup thinly sliced red onion sliced
- ¼ cup snipped fresh cilantro
- 1 tablespoon fresh lime juice
- 2 to 3 tablespoons Jamaican Jerk Seasoning (see recipe)
- 1 tablespoons extra virgin olive oil
- 2 tablespoons avocado oil

1. Thaw shrimp, if frozen. In a medium bowl stir together mango, onion, cilantro, and lime juice.

2. Peel and devein shrimp. Rinse shrimp; pat dry with paper towels. Place shrimp in a medium bowl. Sprinkle with Jamaican Jerk Seasoning; toss to coat shrimp on all sides.

3. In a large nonstick skillet heat olive oil over medium-high heat. Add shrimp; cook and stir about 4 minutes or until opaque. Drizzle shrimp with avocado oil and serve with the mango mixture.

SHRIMP SCAMPI WITH WILTED SPINACH AND RADICCHIO

PREP: 15 minutes COOK: 8 minutes MAKES: 3 servings

"SCAMPI" REFERS TO A CLASSIC RESTAURANT DISH OF LARGE SHRIMP SAUTÉED OR BROILED WITH BUTTER AND LOTS OF GARLIC AND LEMON. THIS SPICY OLIVE OIL VERSION IS PALEO-APPROVED—AND BUMPED UP NUTRITIONALLY WITH A QUICK SAUTÉ OF RADICCHIO AND SPINACH.

- 1 pound fresh or frozen large shrimp
- 4 tablespoons extra virgin olive oil
- 6 cloves garlic, minced
- ½ teaspoon black pepper
- ¼ cup dry white wine
- ½ cup snipped fresh parsley
- ½ of a head radicchio, cored and thinly sliced
- ½ teaspoon crushed red pepper
- 9 cups baby spinach
- Lemon wedges

1. Thaw shrimp, if frozen. Peel and devein shrimp, leaving tails intact. In a large skillet heat 2 tablespoons of the olive oil over medium-high heat. Add shrimp, 4 cloves minced garlic, and black pepper. Cook and stir about 3 minutes or until shrimp are opaque. Transfer shrimp mixture to a bowl.

2. Add white wine to skillet. Cook, stirring to loosen to any browned garlic from bottom of the skillet. Pour wine over shrimp; toss to combine. Stir in parsley. Cover loosely with foil to keep warm; set aside.

3. Add the remaining 2 tablespoons olive oil, the remaining 2 cloves minced garlic, the radicchio, and crushed red pepper to the skillet. Cook and stir over medium heat for 3 minutes or until radicchio just begins to wilt. Carefully stir in the spinach; cook and stir for 1 to 2 minutes more or until spinach is just wilted.

4. To serve, divide spinach mixture among three serving plates; top with shrimp mixture. Serve with lemon wedges for squeezing over shrimp and greens.

CRAB SALAD WITH AVOCADO, GRAPEFRUIT, AND JICAMA

START TO FINISH: 30 minutes MAKES: 4 servings

JUMBO LUMP OR BACKFIN CRABMEAT IS BEST FOR THIS SALAD. JUMBO LUMP CRABMEAT IS MADE UP OF LARGE CHUNKS THAT WORK WELL IN SALADS. BACKFIN IS A BLEND OF BROKEN PIECES OF JUMBO LUMP CRABMEAT AND SMALLER PIECES OF CRABMEAT FROM THE BODY OF THE CRAB. ALTHOUGH SMALLER THAN THE JUMBO LUMP CRAB, BACKFIN WORKS JUST FINE. FRESH IS BEST, OF COURSE, BUT THAWED FROZEN CRAB IS A FINE OPTION.

6 cups baby spinach

½ of a medium jicama, peeled and julienne-cut*

2 pink or ruby red grapefruit, peeled, seeded, and sectioned**

2 small avocados, halved

1 pound jumbo lump or backfin crabmeat

Basil-Grapefruit Dressing (see recipe, right)

1. Divide spinach among four serving plates. Top with jicama, grapefruit sections and any accumulated juice, avocados, and crabmeat. Drizzle with Basil-Grapefruit Dressing.

Basil-Grapefruit Dressing: In a screw-top jar combine ⅓ cup extra virgin olive oil; ¼ cup fresh grapefruit juice; 2 tablespoons fresh orange juice; ½ of a small shallot, minced; 2 tablespoons finely snipped fresh basil; ¼ teaspoon crushed red pepper; and ¼ teaspoon black pepper. Cover and shake well.

*Tip: A julienne peeler makes quick work of cutting the jicama into thin strips.

**Tip: To section grapefruit, cut a slice off the stem end and bottom of the fruit. Set it upright on a work surface. Cut down the fruit in sections from top to bottom, following the rounded shape of the fruit, to remove peel in strips. Hold the fruit over a bowl and, using a paring knife, cut to the center of the fruit on the sides of each segment to release it from the pith. Place segments in bowl with any accumulated juices. Discard pith.

CAJUN LOBSTER TAIL BOIL WITH TARRAGON AÏOLI

PREP: 20 minutes COOK: 30 minutes MAKES: 4 servings PHOTO

FOR A ROMANTIC DINNER FOR TWO, THIS RECIPE IS EASILY CUT IN HALF. USE VERY SHARP KITCHEN SHEARS TO CUT OPEN THE SHELL OF THE LOBSTER TAILS AND GET AT THE RICHLY FLAVORED MEAT.

- 2 recipes Cajun Seasoning (see recipe)
- 12 cloves garlic, peeled and halved
- 2 lemons, halved
- 2 large carrots, peeled
- 2 celery stalks, peeled
- 2 fennel bulbs, sliced into thin wedges
- 1 pound whole button mushrooms
- 4 7- to 8-ounce Maine lobster tails
- 4 8-inch bamboo skewers
- ½ cup Paleo Aïoli (Garlic Mayo) (see recipe)
- ¼ cup Dijon-Style Mustard (see recipe)
- 2 tablespoons snipped fresh tarragon or parsley

1. In an 8-quart stockpot combine 6 cups water, Cajun Seasoning, garlic, and lemons. Bring to boiling; boil for 5 minutes. Reduce heat to keep liquid at a simmer.

2. Cut the carrots and celery crosswise into four pieces. Add carrots, celery, and fennel to liquid. Cover and cook for 10 minutes. Add mushrooms; cover and cook for 5 minutes. Using a slotted spoon, transfer vegetables to a serving bowl; keep warm.

3. Starting from the body end of each lobster tail, slide a skewer between the meat and the shell, going almost all the way through the tail end. (This will keep the tail from curling as it cooks.) Reduce heat. Cook lobster tails in the barely simmering liquid in pot for 8 to 12 minutes or until shells turn bright red and meat is tender when pierced with a fork. Remove lobster from cooking liquid. Use a kitchen towel to hold the lobster tails and remove and discard the skewers.

4. In a small bowl stir together the Paleo Aïoli, Dijon-Style Mustard, and tarragon. Serve with the lobster and vegetables.

MUSSELS FRITES WITH SAFFRON AÏOLI

START TO FINISH: 1¼ hours MAKES: 4 servings

THIS IS A PALEO TAKE ON THE FRENCH CLASSIC OF MUSSELS STEAMED IN WHITE WINE AND HERBS AND SERVED WITH THIN AND CRISPY FRITES MADE FROM WHITE POTATOES. DISCARD ANY MUSSELS THAT WON'T CLOSE BEFORE THEY'RE COOKED—AND ANY MUSSELS THAT DON'T OPEN AFTER THEY'RE COOKED.

PARSNIP FRITES

- 1½ pounds parsnips, peeled and cut into 3×¼-inch julienne
- 3 tablespoons olive oil
- 2 cloves garlic, minced
- ¼ teaspoon black pepper
- ⅛ teaspoon cayenne pepper

SAFFRON AÏOLI

- ⅓ cup Paleo Aïoli (Garlic Mayo) (see recipe)
- ⅛ teaspoon saffron threads, gently crushed

MUSSELS

- 4 tablespoons olive oil
- ½ cup finely chopped shallots
- 6 cloves garlic, minced
- ¼ teaspoon black pepper
- 3 cups dry white wine
- 3 large sprigs flat-leaf parsley
- 4 pounds mussels, cleaned and debearded*
- ¼ cup chopped fresh Italian (flat-leaf) parsley
- 2 tablespoons snipped fresh tarragon (optional)

1. For parsnip frites, preheat oven to 450°F. Soak cut parsnips in enough cold water to cover in the refrigerator for 30 minutes; drain and pat dry with paper towels.

2. Line a large baking sheet with parchment paper. Place parsnips in an extra-large bowl. In a small bowl combine 3 tablespoons olive oil, 2 cloves minced garlic, ¼ teaspoon black pepper, and cayenne pepper; drizzle over parsnips and toss to coat. Arrange parsnips in an even layer on prepared baking sheet. Bake for 30 to 35 minutes or tender and starting to brown, stirring occasionally.

3. For aïoli, in a small bowl stir together Paleo Aïoli and saffron. Cover and refrigerate until serving time.

4. Meanwhile, in a 6- to 8-quart stockpot or Dutch oven heat the 4 tablespoons olive oil over medium heat. Add shallots, 6 cloves garlic, and ¼ teaspoon black pepper; cook about 2 minutes or until soft and wilted, stirring frequently.

5. Add wine and parsley sprigs to pot; bring to boiling. Add mussels, stirring a few times. Cover tightly and steam for 3 to 5 minutes or until shells open, gently stirring twice. Discard any mussels that do not open.

6. With a large skimmer, transfer mussels into shallow soup dishes. Remove and discard parsley sprigs from cooking liquid; ladle cooking liquid over the mussels. Sprinkle with chopped parsley and, if desired, tarragon. Serve immediately with parsnip frites and saffron aïoli.

*Tip: Cook mussels the day they are purchased. If using wild-harvested mussels, soak in a bowl of cold water for 20 minutes to help flush out grit and sand. (This is not necessary for farm-raised mussels.) Using a stiff brush, scrub mussels, one at a time, under cold running water. Debeard mussels about 10 to 15 minutes before cooking. The beard is the small cluster of fibers that emerge from the shell. To remove the beards, grasp the string between your thumb and forefinger and yank toward the hinge. (This method will not kill the mussel.) You can also use pliers or fish tweezers. Be sure that the shell of each mussel is tightly closed. If any shells are open, tap them gently on the counter. Discard any mussels that don't close within a few minutes. Discard any mussels with cracked or damaged shells.

SEARED SCALLOPS WITH BEET RELISH

START TO FINISH: 30 minutes MAKES: 4 servings PHOTO

FOR A BEAUTIFUL GOLDEN CRUST, BE SURE THE SURFACE OF THE SCALLOPS IS REALLY DRY—AND THAT THE PAN IS NICE AND HOT—BEFORE ADDING THEM TO THE PAN. ALSO, LET THE SCALLOPS SEAR WITHOUT DISTURBING THEM FOR 2 TO 3 MINUTES, CAREFULLY CHECKING BEFORE TURNING.

1 pound fresh or frozen sea scallops, patted dry with paper towels
3 medium red beets, peeled and cut chopped
½ of a Granny Smith apple, peeled and chopped
2 jalapeños, stemmed, seeded, and minced (see tip)
¼ cup chopped fresh cilantro
2 tablespoons finely chopped red onion
4 tablespoons olive oil
2 tablespoons fresh lime juice
White pepper

1. Thaw scallops, if frozen.

2. For beet relish, in a medium bowl combine beets, apple, jalapeños, cilantro, onion, 2 tablespoons of the olive oil, and lime juice. Mix well. Set aside while preparing scallops.

3. Rinse scallops; pat dry with paper towels. In a large skillet heat the remaining 2 tablespoons olive oil over medium-high heat. Add scallops; sauté for 4 to 6 minutes or until golden brown on the exterior and barely opaque. Sprinkle scallops lightly with white pepper.

4. To serve, divide beet relish evenly among serving plates; top with scallops. Serve immediately.

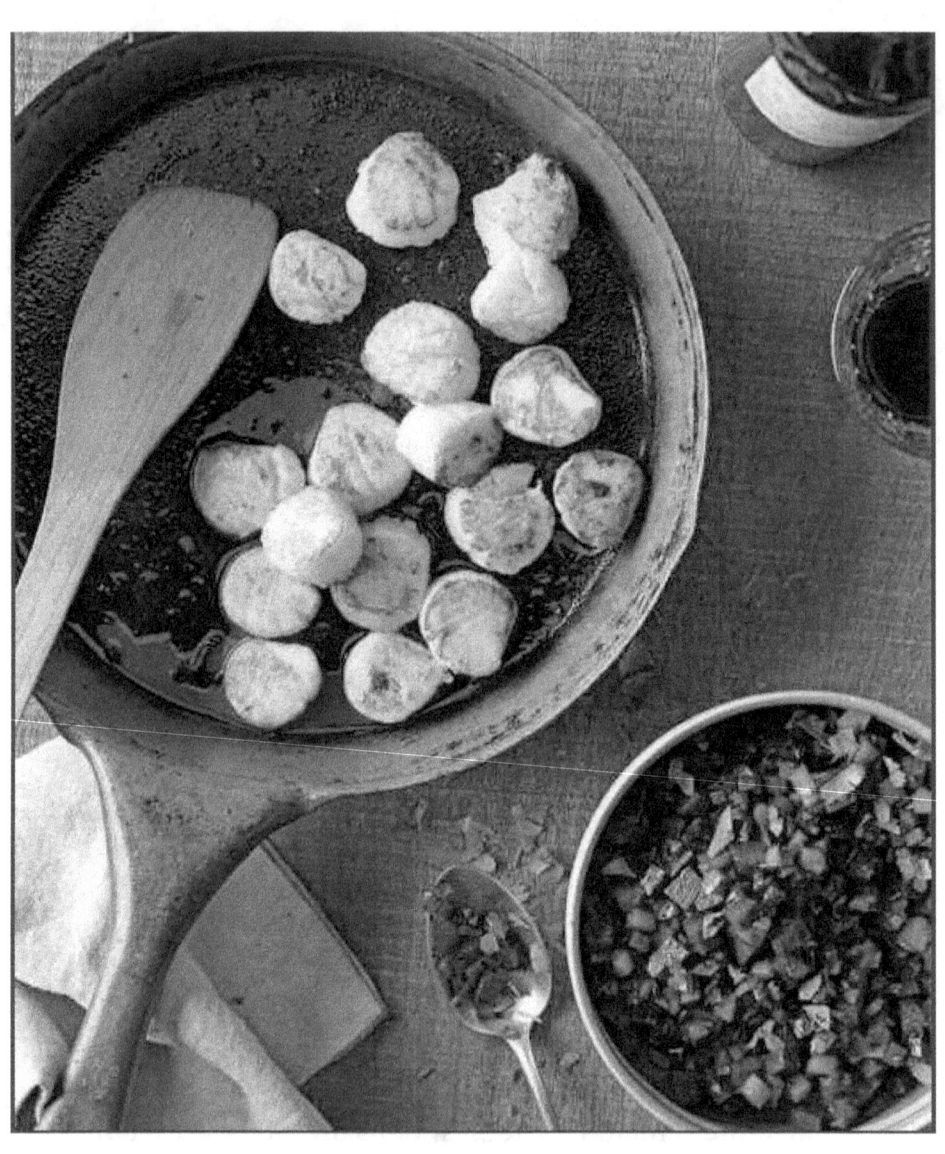

GRILLED SCALLOPS WITH CUCUMBER-DILL SALSA

PREP: 35 minutes CHILL: 1 to 24 hours GRILL: 9 minutes MAKES: 4 servings

HERE'S A TIP FOR GETTING THE MOST FLAWLESS AVOCADOS: BUY THEM WHEN THEY ARE BRIGHT GREEN AND HARD, THEN RIPEN THEM ON THE COUNTER FOR A FEW DAYS—UNTIL THEY GIVE JUST SLIGHTLY WHEN LIGHTLY PRESSED WITH YOUR FINGERS. WHEN HARD AND UNRIPE, THEY WON'T BRUISE IN TRANSIT FROM THE MARKET.

12 or 16 fresh or frozen sea scallops (1¼ to 1¾ pounds total)

¼ cup olive oil

4 cloves garlic, minced

1 teaspoon freshly ground black pepper

2 medium zucchini, trimmed and halved lengthwise

½ of a medium cucumber, halved lengthwise and thinly sliced crosswise

1 medium avocado, halved, seeded, peeled, and chopped

1 medium tomato, cored, seeded, and chopped

2 teaspoons snipped fresh mint

1 teaspoon snipped fresh dill

1. Thaw scallops, if frozen. Rinse scallops with cold water; pat dry with paper towels. In a large bowl combine 3 tablespoons of the oil, the garlic, and ¾ teaspoon of the pepper. Add scallops; toss gently to coat. Cover and chill for at least 1 hour or up to 24 hours, gently stirring occasionally.

2. Brush zucchini halves with the remaining 1 tablespoon oil; sprinkle evenly with remaining ¼ teaspoon pepper.

3. Drain scallops, discarding marinade. Thread two 10- to 12-inch skewers through each scallop, using 3 or 4 scallops for each pair of skewers and leaving a ½-inch space between scallops.* (Threading the scallops on two skewers helps keep them stable when grilling and turning.)

4. For a charcoal or gas grill, place scallop kabobs and zucchini halves on the grill rack directly over medium heat.** Cover and grill until scallops are opaque and zucchini are just tender, turning halfway through grilling. Allow 6 to 8 minutes for scallops and 9 to 11 minutes for zucchini.

5. Meanwhile, for salsa, in a medium bowl combine cucumber, avocado, tomato, mint, and dill. Toss gently to combine. Place 1 scallop kabob on each of four serving plates. Diagonally cut zucchini halves crosswise in half and add to plates with scallops. Spoon cucumber mixture evenly over scallops.

*Tip: If using wooden skewers, soak in enough water to cover for 30 minutes before using.

**To broil: Prepare as directed through Step 3. Place scallop kabobs and zucchini halves on the unheated rack of a broiler pan. Broil 4 to 5 inches from the heat until scallops are opaque and zucchini is just tender, turning once halfway through cooking. Allow 6 to 8 minutes for scallops and 10 to 12 minutes for zucchini.

SEARED SCALLOPS WITH TOMATO, OLIVE OIL, AND HERB SAUCE

PREP: 20 minutes COOK: 4 minutes MAKES: 4 servings

THE SAUCE IS ALMOST LIKE A WARM VINAIGRETTE. OLIVE OIL, CHOPPED FRESH TOMATO, LEMON JUICE, AND HERBS ARE COMBINED AND VERY GENTLY HEATED—JUST ENOUGH TO MELD THE FLAVORS—AND THEN SERVED WITH THE SEARED SCALLOPS AND A CRUNCHY SUNFLOWER SPROUT SALAD.

SCALLOPS AND SAUCE

    1 to 1½ pounds large fresh or frozen sea scallops (about 12)

    2 large roma tomatoes, peeled,* seeded, and chopped

    ½ cup olive oil

    2 tablespoons fresh lemon juice

    2 tablespoons snipped fresh basil

    1 to 2 teaspoons finely chopped chives

    1 tablespoon olive oil

SALAD

    4 cups sunflower sprouts

    1 lemon, cut into wedges

    Extra virgin olive oil

1. Thaw scallops, if frozen. Rinse scallops; pat dry. Set aside.

2. For sauce, in a small saucepan combine tomatoes, ½ cup olive oil, the lemon juice, basil, and chives; set aside.

3. In a large skillet heat the 1 tablespoon olive oil over medium-high heat. Add scallops; cook for 4 to 5 minutes or until browned and opaque, turning once halfway through cooking.

4. For the salad, place the sprouts in a serving bowl. Squeeze lemon wedges over sprouts and drizzle with a little olive oil. Toss to combine.

5. Heat the sauce over low heat until warm; do not boil. To serve, spoon some of the sauce in the center of the plate; top with 3 of the scallops. Serve with the sprouts salad.

*Tip: To easily peel a tomato, drop the tomato into a pot of boiling water for 30 seconds to 1 minute or until the skin starts to split. Remove tomato from the boiling water and immediately plunge into a bowl of ice water to stop the cooking process. When tomato is cool enough to handle, slip the skin off.

CUMIN-ROASTED CAULIFLOWER WITH FENNEL AND PEARL ONIONS

PREP: 15 minutes COOK: 25 minutes MAKES: 4 servings PHOTO

THERE IS SOMETHING PARTICULARLY ENTICING ABOUT THE COMBINATION OF ROASTED CAULIFLOWER AND THE TOASTY, EARTHY TASTE OF CUMIN. THIS DISH HAS THE ADDITIONAL ELEMENT OF SWEETNESS FROM DRIED CURRANTS. IF YOU LIKE, YOU COULD ADD A LITTLE HEAT WITH ¼ TO ½ TEASPOON OF CRUSHED RED PEPPER ALONG WITH THE CUMIN AND CURRANTS IN STEP 2.

- 3 tablespoons unrefined coconut oil
- 1 medium head cauliflower, cut into florets (4 to 5 cups)
- 2 heads fennel, coarsely chopped
- 1½ cups frozen pearl onions, thawed and drained
- ¼ cup dried currants
- 2 teaspoons ground cumin
- Snipped fresh dill (optional)

1. In an extra-large skillet heat coconut oil over medium heat. Add cauliflower, fennel, and pearl onions. Cover and cook for 15 minutes, stirring occasionally.

2. Reduce heat to medium-low. Add currants and cumin to skillet; cook, uncovered, about 10 minutes or until cauliflower and fennel are tender and golden brown. If desired, garnish with dill.

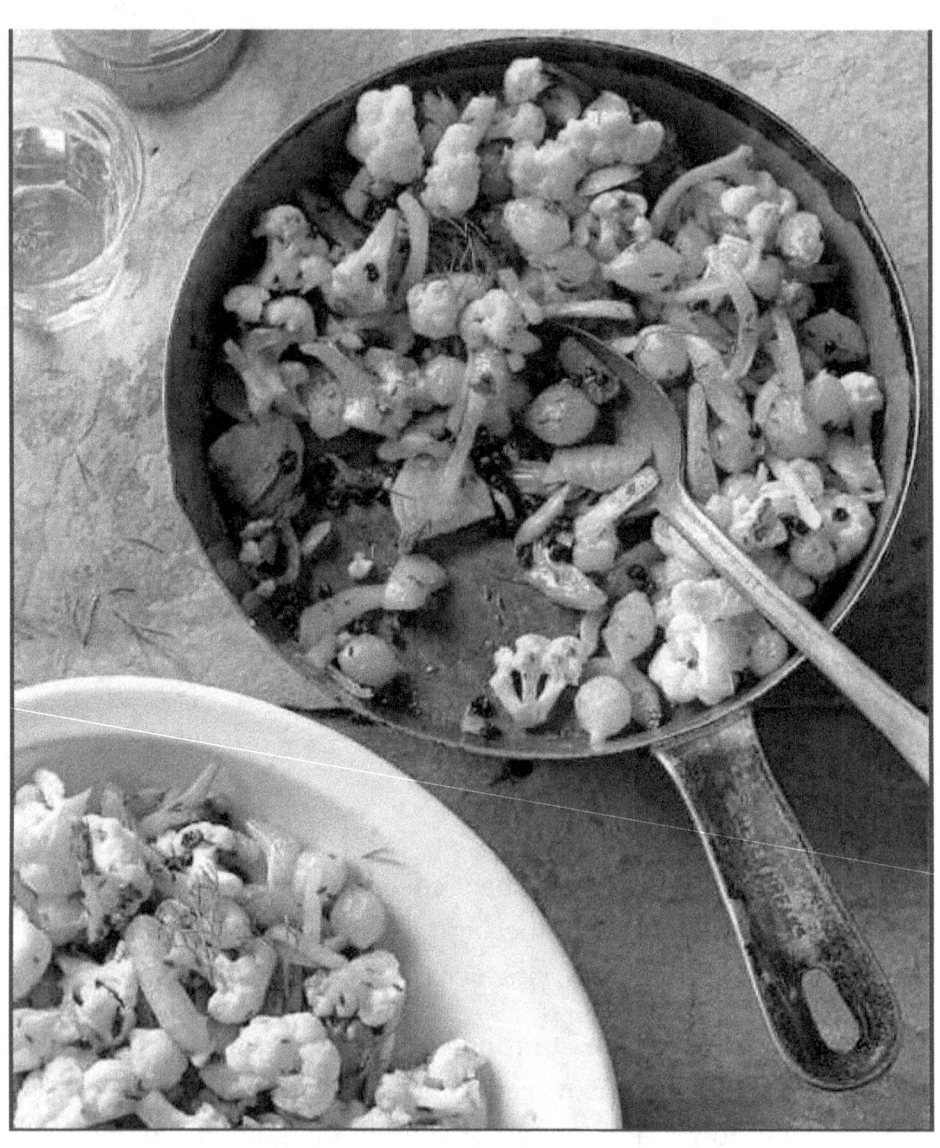

CHUNKY TOMATO-EGGPLANT SAUCE WITH SPAGHETTI SQUASH

PREP: 30 minutes BAKE: 50 minutes COOL: 10 minutes COOK: 10 minutes MAKES: 4 servings

THIS SAUCY SIDE DISH IS EASILY TURNED INTO A MAIN DISH. ADD ABOUT 1 POUND OF COOKED GROUND BEEF OR BISON TO THE EGGPLANT-TOMATO MIXTURE AFTER YOU MASH IT LIGHTLY WITH A POTATO MASHER.

1 2- to 2½-pound spaghetti squash
2 tablespoons olive oil
1 cup chopped, peeled eggplant
¾ cup chopped onion
1 small red sweet pepper, chopped (½ cup)
4 cloves garlic, minced
4 medium red ripe tomatoes, peeled if desired and coarsely chopped (about 2 cups)
½ cup torn fresh basil

1. Preheat oven to 375°F. Line a small baking pan with parchment paper. Cut spaghetti squash in half crosswise. Use a large spoon to scrape out any seeds and strings. Place squash halves, cut sides down, on prepared baking sheet. Bake, uncovered, for 50 to 60 minutes or until squash is tender. Cool on a wire rack about 10 minutes.

2. Meanwhile, in a large skillet heat olive oil over medium heat. Add onion, eggplant and pepper; cook for 5 to 7 minutes or until vegetables are tender, stirring occasionally. Add garlic; cook and stir 30 seconds more. Add tomatoes; cook for 3 to 5 minutes or until tomatoes are softened, stirring occasionally. Using a potato masher,

mash the mixture lightly. Stir in half the basil. Cover and cook for 2 minutes.

3. Use a pot holder or towel to hold squash halves. Use a fork to scrape the squash pulp into a medium bowl. Divide squash among four serving plates. Top evenly with sauce. Sprinkle with remaining basil.

STUFFED PORTOBELLO MUSHROOMS

PREP: 35 minutes BAKE: 20 minutes COOK: 7 minutes MAKES: 4 servings

TO GET THE FRESHEST PORTOBELLOS, LOOK FOR MUSHROOMS THAT STILL HAVE THEIR STEMS INTACT. THE GILLS SHOULD LOOK MOIST BUT NOT WET OR BLACK AND SHOULD HAVE GOOD SEPARATION BETWEEN THEM. TO PREPARE ANY KIND OF MUSHROOMS FOR COOKING, WIPE WITH A SLIGHTLY DAMP PAPER TOWEL. NEVER RUN MUSHROOMS UNDER WATER OR SOAK THEM IN WATER—THEY ARE HIGHLY ABSORBENT AND WILL GET MUSHY AND WATERLOGGED.

4 large portobello mushrooms (about 1 pound total)
¼ cup olive oil
1 tablespoon Smoky Seasoning (see recipe)
2 tablespoons olive oil
½ cup chopped shallots
1 tablespoon minced garlic
1 pound Swiss chard, stemmed and chopped (about 10 cups)
2 teaspoons Mediterranean Seasoning (see recipe)
½ cup chopped radishes

1. Preheat oven to 400°F. Remove stems from mushrooms and reserve for Step 2. Use the tip of a spoon to scrape the gills out of the caps; discard gills. Place mushroom caps in a 3-quart rectangular baking dish; brush both sides of mushrooms with the ¼ cup olive oil. Turn mushroom caps so the stemmed sides are up; sprinkle with Smoky Seasoning. Cover baking dish with foil. Bake, covered, about 20 minutes or until tender.

2. Meanwhile, chop reserved mushroom stems; set aside. To prepare chard, remove thick ribs from leaves and discard. Coarsely chop the chard leaves.

3. In an extra-large skillet heat the 2 tablespoons olive oil over medium heat. Add shallots and garlic; cook and stir for 30 seconds. Add chopped mushroom stems, chopped chard, and Mediterranean Seasoning. Cook, uncovered, for 6 to 8 minutes or until chard is tender, stirring occasionally.

4. Divide chard mixture among the mushroom caps. Drizzle any liquid remaining in baking dish over stuffed mushrooms. Top with chopped radishes.

ROASTED RADICCHIO

PREP: 20 minutes COOK: 15 minutes MAKES: 4 servings

RADICCHIO IS MOST OFTEN EATEN AS PART OF A SALAD TO PROVIDE A PLEASANT BITTERNESS AMONG THE MIX OF GREENS—BUT IT CAN BE ROASTED OR GRILLED ON ITS OWN AS WELL. A SLIGHT BITTERNESS IS INHERENT TO RADICCHIO, BUT YOU DON'T WANT IT TO BE OVERWHELMING. LOOK FOR SMALLER HEADS WHOSE LEAVES LOOK FRESH AND CRISP—NOT WILTED. THE CUT END MAY BE A LITTLE BROWN BUT SHOULD BE MOSTLY WHITE. IN THIS RECIPE, A SPLASH OF BALSAMIC VINEGAR BEFORE SERVING ADDS A HINT OF SWEETNESS.

2 large heads radicchio

¼ cup olive oil

1 teaspoon Mediterranean Seasoning (see recipe)

¼ cup balsamic vinegar

1. Preheat oven to 400°F. Quarter the radicchio, leaving some of the core attached (you should have 8 wedges). Brush cut sides of radicchio wedges with olive oil. Place wedges, cut sides down, on a baking sheet; sprinkle with Mediterranean Seasoning.

2. Roast about 15 minutes or until radicchio wilts, turning once halfway through roasting. Arrange radicchio on a serving platter. Drizzle balsamic vinegar; serve immediately.

ROASTED FENNEL WITH ORANGE VINAIGRETTE

PREP: 25 minutes ROAST: 25 minutes MAKES: 4 servings

SAVE ANY LEFTOVER VINAIGRETTE TO TOSS WITH SALAD GREENS—OR SERVE WITH GRILLED PORK, POULTRY, OR FISH. STORE LEFTOVER VINAIGRETTE IN A TIGHTLY COVERED CONTAINER IN THE REFRIGERATOR FOR UP TO 3 DAYS.

- 6 tablespoons extra virgin olive oil, plus more for brushing
- 1 large fennel bulb, trimmed, cored, and cut into wedges (reserve fronds for garnish if desired)
- 1 red onion, cut into wedges
- ½ of an orange, thinly sliced into rounds
- ½ cup orange juice
- 2 tablespoons white wine vinegar or champagne vinegar
- 2 tablespoons apple cider
- 1 teaspoon ground fennel seeds
- 1 teaspoon finely shredded orange peel
- ½ teaspoon Dijon-Style Mustard (see recipe)
- Black pepper

1. Preheat oven to 425°F. Brush a large baking sheet lightly with olive oil. Arrange the fennel, onion, and orange slices on the baking sheet; drizzle with 2 tablespoons of the olive oil. Gently toss vegetable to coat with oil.

2. Roast vegetables for 25 to 30 minutes or until vegetables are tender and light golden, turning once halfway through roasting.

3. Meanwhile, for orange vinaigrette, in a blender combine orange juice, vinegar, apple cider, fennel seeds, orange

peel, Dijon-Style Mustard, and pepper to taste. With the blender running, slowly add the remaining 4 tablespoons olive oil in a thin stream. Continue blending until vinaigrette thickens.

4. Transfer vegetables to a serving platter. Drizzle vegetables with some of the vinaigrette. If desired, garnish with reserved fennel fronds.

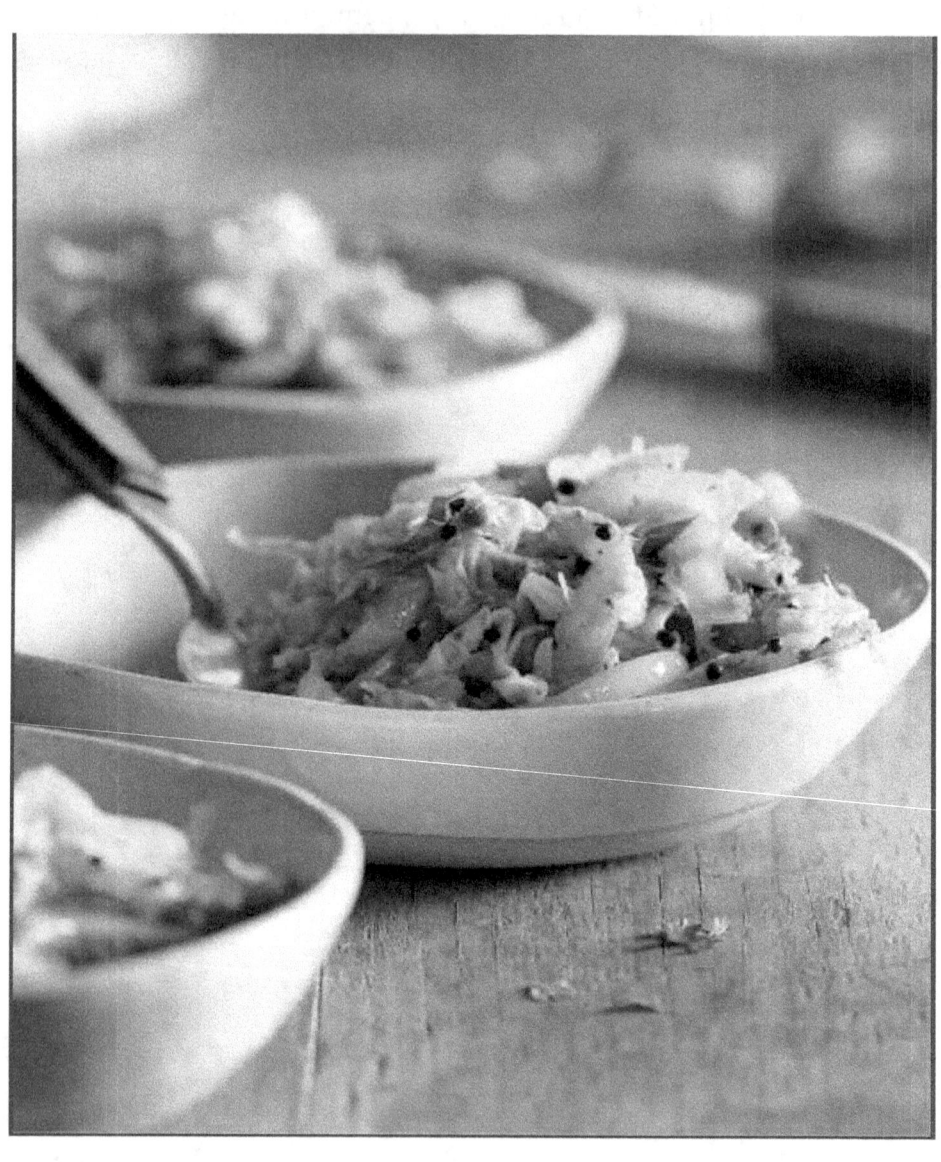

PUNJABI-STYLE SAVOY CABBAGE

PREP: 20 minutes COOK: 25 minutes MAKES: 4 servings PHOTO

IT'S AMAZING WHAT HAPPENS TO A MILDLY-FLAVORED, UNASSUMING CABBAGE WHEN IT'S COOKED WITH GINGER, GARLIC, CHILES, AND INDIAN SPICES. TOASTED MUSTARD, CORIANDER, AND CUMIN SEEDS GIVE THIS DISH BOTH FLAVOR AND CRUNCH. BE FOREWARNED: IT IS HOT! BIRD'S BEAK CHILES ARE SMALL BUT VERY POTENT—AND THE DISH INCLUDES JALAPEÑO TOO. IF YOU PREFER LESS HEAT, JUST USE THE JALAPEÑO.

- 1 2-inch knob fresh ginger, peeled and cut into ⅓-inch slices
- 5 cloves garlic
- 1 large jalapeño, stemmed, seeded, and halved (see tip)
- 2 teaspoons no-salt-added garam masala
- 1 teaspoon ground turmeric
- ½ cup Chicken Bone Broth (see recipe) or no-salt-added chicken broth
- 3 tablespoons refined coconut oil
- 1 tablespoon black mustard seeds
- 1 teaspoon coriander seeds
- 1 teaspoon cumin seeds
- 1 whole bird's beak chile (chile de arbol) (see tip)
- 1 3-inch cinnamon stick
- 2 cups thinly sliced yellow onions (about 2 medium)
- 12 cups thinly sliced, cored savoy cabbage (about 1½ pounds)
- ½ cup snipped fresh cilantro (optional)

1. In a food processor or blender combine ginger, garlic, jalapeño, garam masala, turmeric, and ¼ cup of the Chicken Bone Broth. Cover and process or blend until smooth; set aside.

2. In an extra-large skillet combine coconut oil, mustard seeds, coriander seeds, cumin seeds, chile, and cinnamon stick. Cook over medium-high heat, shaking pan frequently, for 2 to 3 minutes or until the cinnamon stick unfurls.(Be careful—mustard seeds will pop and spatter as they cook.) Add onions; cook and stir for 5 to 6 minutes or until onions are lightly browned. Add ginger mixture. Cook, for 6 to 8 minutes or until mixture is nicely caramelized, stirring often.

3. Add cabbage and the remaining Chicken Bone Broth; mix well. Cover and cook about 15 minutes or until cabbage is tender, stirring twice. Uncover skillet. Cook and stir for 6 to 7 minutes or until cabbage is lightly browned and excess Chicken Bone Broth evaporates.

4. Remove and discard cinnamon stick and chile. If desired, sprinkle with cilantro.

CINNAMON-ROASTED BUTTERNUT SQUASH

PREP: 20 minutes ROAST: 30 minutes MAKES: 4 to 6 servings

A DASH OF CAYENNE PEPPER GIVES THESE SWEET ROASTED CUBES OF SQUASH JUST A HINT OF HEAT. IT'S EASILY LEFT OUT IF YOU PREFER. SERVE THIS SIMPLE SIDE WITH ROAST PORK OR PORK CHOPS.

- 1 butternut squash (about 2 pounds), peeled, seeded, and cut into ¾-inch cubes
- 2 tablespoons olive oil
- ½ teaspoon ground cinnamon
- ¼ teaspoon black pepper
- ⅛ teaspoon cayenne pepper

1. Preheat oven to 400°F. In a large bowl toss squash with olive oil, cinnamon, black pepper, and cayenne pepper. Line a large rimmed baking sheet with parchment paper. Spread squash in a single layer on the baking sheet.

2. Roast for 30 to 35 minutes or until squash is tender and browned on edges, stirring once or twice.

BROILED ASPARAGUS WITH SIEVED EGG AND PECANS

START TO FINISH: 15 minutes MAKES: 4 servings

THIS IS A TAKE ON A CLASSIC FRENCH VEGETABLE DISH CALLED ASPARAGUS MIMOSA—SO CALLED BECAUSE THE GREEN, WHITE, AND YELLOW OF THE FINISHED DISH LOOKS LIKE A FLOWER OF THE SAME NAME.

- 1 pound fresh asparagus, trimmed
- 5 tablespoons Roasted Garlic Vinaigrette (see recipe)
- 1 hard-cooked egg, peeled
- 3 tablespoons chopped pecans, toasted (see tip)
- Freshly ground black pepper

1. Position oven rack 4 inches from heating element; preheat broiler to high.

2. Spread asparagus spears on a baking sheet. Drizzle with 2 tablespoons of the Roasted Garlic Vinaigrette. Using your hands, roll asparagus to coat with vinaigrette. Broil for 3 to 5 minutes or until blistered and tender, turning asparagus after every minute. Transfer to a serving platter.

3. Cut the egg in half; press egg through a sieve over the asparagus. (You can also grate the egg using the large holes of a box grater.) Drizzle asparagus and egg with the remaining 3 tablespoons Roasted Garlic Vinaigrette. Top with pecans and sprinkle with pepper.

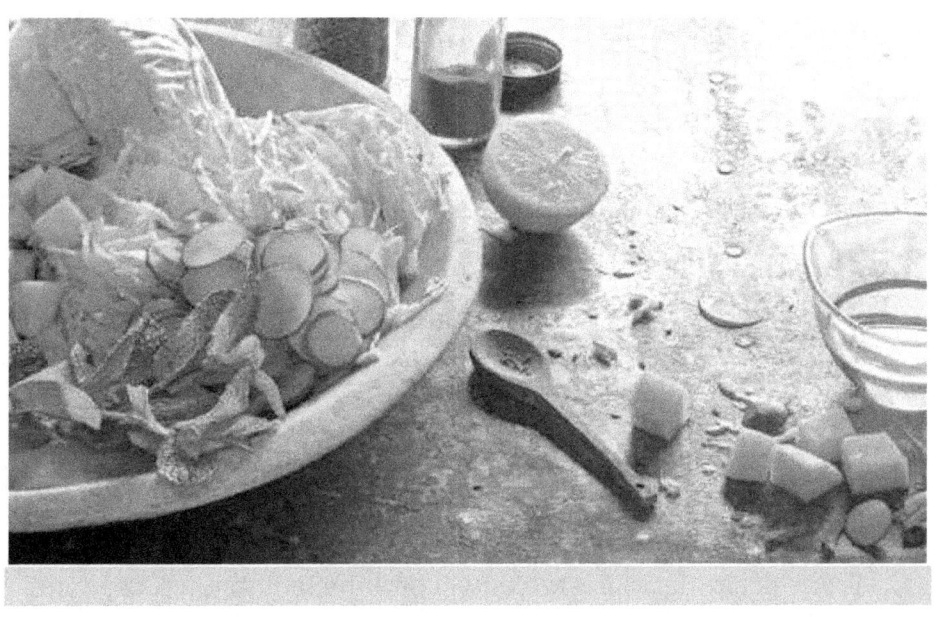

CRUNCHY CABBAGE SLAW WITH RADISHES, MANGO, AND MINT

START TO FINISH: 20 minutes MAKES: 6 servings PHOTO

3 tablespoons fresh lemon juice

¼ teaspoon cayenne pepper

¼ teaspoon ground cumin

¼ cup olive oil

4 cups shredded cabbage

1½ cups very thinly sliced radishes

1 cup cubed ripe mango

½ cup bias-sliced scallions

⅓ cup chopped fresh mint

1. For dressing, in a large bowl combine lemon juice, cayenne pepper, and ground cumin. Whisk in olive oil in a thin stream.

2. Add cabbage, radishes, mango, scallions, and mint to dressing in bowl. Toss well to combine.

ROASTED CABBAGE ROUNDS WITH CARAWAY AND LEMON

PREP: 10 minutes ROAST: 30 minutes MAKES: 4 to 6 servings

3 tablespoons olive oil
1 medium head cabbage, cut into 1-inch-thick rounds
2 teaspoons Dijon-Style Mustard (see recipe)
1 teaspoon finely shredded lemon peel
¼ teaspoon black pepper
1 teaspoon caraway seeds
Lemon wedges

1. Preheat oven to 400°F. Brush a large rimmed baking sheet with 1 tablespoon of the olive oil. Arrange cabbage rounds on the baking sheet; set aside.

2. In a small bowl whisk together the remaining 2 tablespoons olive oil, Dijon-Style Mustard, and lemon peel. Brush over cabbage rounds on baking sheet, making sure mustard and lemon peel are evenly distributed. Sprinkle with pepper and caraway seeds.

3. Roast for 30 to 35 minutes or until cabbage is tender and edges are golden brown. Serve with lemon wedges to squeeze over cabbage.

ROASTED CABBAGE WITH ORANGE-BALSAMIC DRIZZLE

PREP: 15 minutes ROAST: 30 minutes MAKES: 4 servings

3 tablespoons olive oil
1 small head cabbage, cored and cut into 8 wedges
½ teaspoon black pepper
⅓ cup balsamic vinegar
2 teaspoons finely shredded orange peel

1. Preheat oven to 450°F. Brush a large rimmed baking sheet with 1 tablespoon of the olive oil. Arrange cabbage wedges on the baking sheet. Brush cabbage with the remaining 2 tablespoons olive oil and sprinkle with pepper.

2. Roast cabbage for 15 minutes. Turn cabbage wedges over; roast about 15 minutes more or until cabbage is tender and edges are golden brown.

3. In a small saucepan combine the balsamic vinegar and orange peel. Bring to boiling over medium heat; reduce. Simmer, uncovered, about 4 minutes or until reduced by half. Drizzle over roasted cabbage wedges; serve immediately.

BRAISED CABBAGE WITH CREAMY DILL SAUCE AND TOASTED WALNUTS

PREP: 20 minutes COOK: 40 minutes MAKES: 6 servings

3 tablespoons olive oil
1 shallot, finely chopped
1 small head green cabbage, cut into 6 wedges
½ teaspoon black pepper
1 cup Chicken Bone Broth (see recipe) or no-salt-added chicken broth
¾ cup Cashew Cream (see recipe)
4 teaspoons finely shredded lemon peel
4 teaspoons snipped fresh dill
1 tablespoon finely chopped scallions
¼ cup chopped walnuts, toasted (see tip)

1. In an extra-large skillet heat olive oil over medium-high heat. Add shallot; cook for 2 to 3 minutes or until tender and lightly browned. Add cabbage wedges to skillet. Cook, uncovered, for 10 minutes or until lightly browned on each side, turning once halfway through cooking. Sprinkle with pepper.

2. Add Chicken Bone Broth to skillet. Bring to boiling; reduce heat. Cover and simmer for 25 to 30 minutes or until cabbage is tender.

3. Meanwhile, for Creamy Dill Sauce, in a small bowl stir together Cashew Cream, lemon peel, dill, and scallions.

4. To serve, transfer cabbage wedges to serving plates; drizzle with pan juices. Top with dill sauce and sprinkle with toasted walnuts.

SAUTÉED GREEN CABBAGE WITH TOASTED SESAME SEEDS

PREP: 20 minutes COOK: 19 minutes MAKES: 4 servings

2 tablespoons sesame seeds
2 tablespoons refined coconut oil
1 medium onion, thinly sliced
1 medium tomato, chopped
1 tablespoon minced fresh ginger
3 cloves garlic, minced
¼ teaspoon crushed red pepper
½ of a 3- to 3½-pound head green cabbage, cored and very thinly sliced

1. In an extra-large dry skillet toast sesame seeds over medium heat for 3 to 4 minutes or until golden brown, stirring almost constantly. Transfer seeds to a smal bowl and cool completely. Transfer seeds to a clean spice or coffee grinder; pulse to grind coarsely. Set ground sesame seeds aside.

2. Meanwhile, in the same extra-large skillet heat coconut oil over medium-high heat. Add onion; cook about 2 minutes or just until slightly soft. Stir in tomato, ginger, garlic, and crushed red pepper. Cook and stir for 2 minutes more.

3. Add sliced cabbage to tomato mixture in skillet. Toss with tongs to combine. Cook for 12 to 14 minutes or until cabbage is tender and just begins to brown, stirring occasionally. Add ground sesame seeds; stir well to combine. Serve immediately.

www.ingramcontent.com/pod-product-compliance
Lightning Source LLC
Chambersburg PA
CBHW071823080526

44589CB00012B/901